S0-BXY-380

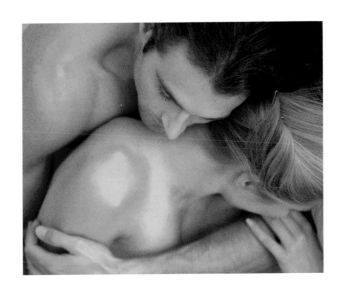

tantricsex
the path to sexual bliss

kavida rei

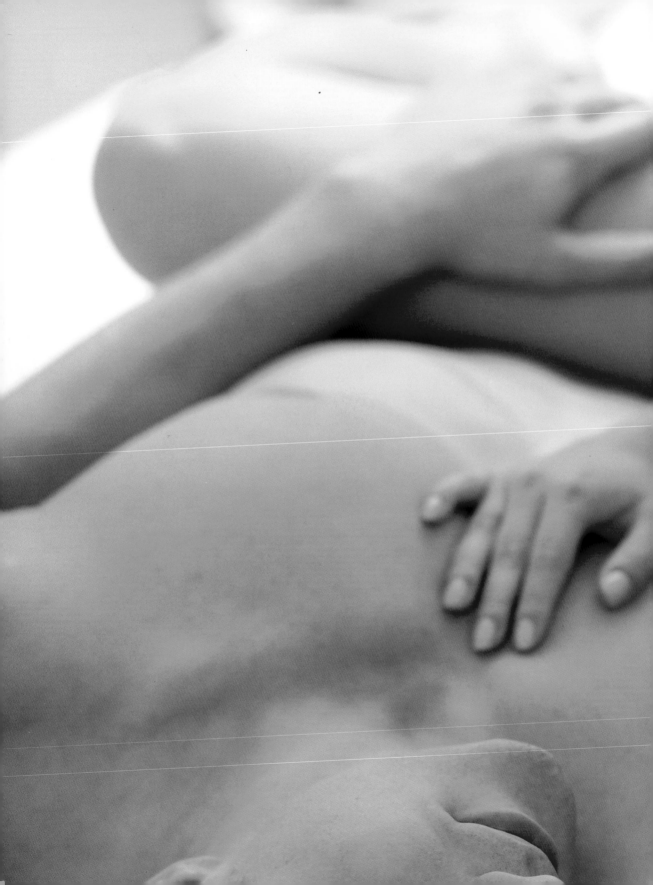

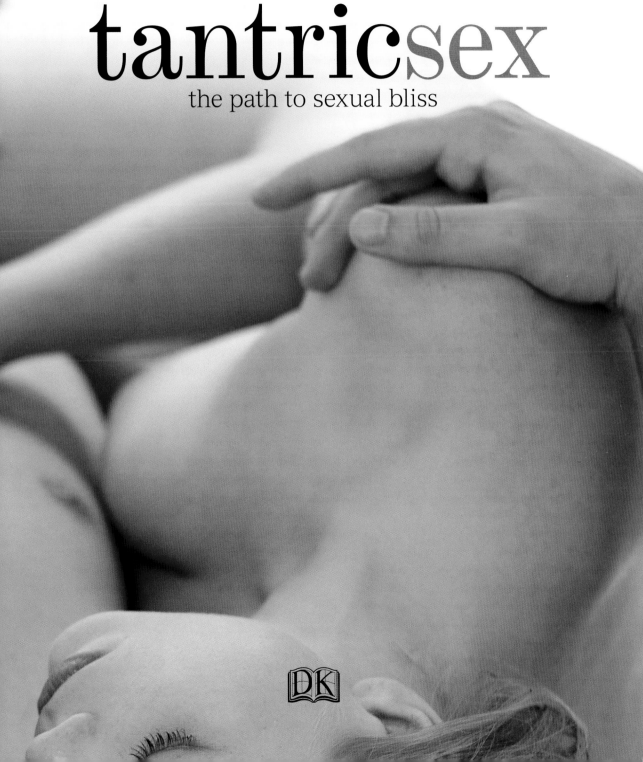

kavida rei

tantric sex

the path to sexual bliss

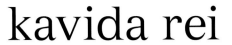

London, New York, Melbourne, Munich, and Delhi

Editor: Nichole Morford
Senior Art Editor: Helen Spencer
Project Art Editor: Natasha Montgomery
Executive Managing Editor: Adèle Hayward
Managing Art Editor: Kat Mead
Production Editor: Ben Marcus
US Editor: Charles Wills
Creative Technical Support: Sonia Charbonnier
Production Controller: Bethan Blasé
Art Director: Peter Luff
Publisher: Stephanie Jackson

Project Editor: Becky Alexander
Designer: XAB Design

First American Edition, 2008

Published in the United States by
DK Publishing
375 Hudson Street
New York, New York 10014

08 09 10 11   10 9 8 7 6 5 4 3 2 1

TD396—December 2008

Copyright © 2008 Dorling Kindersley Limited
All rights reserved

Without limiting the rights under copyright reserved above,
no part of this publication may be reproduced, stored in or
introduced into a retrieval system, or transmitted, in any form,
or by any means (electronic, mechanical, photocopying,
recording, or otherwise), without the prior written permission
of both the copyright owner and the above publisher of
this book.

Published in Great Britain by Dorling Kindersley Limited.

A catalog record for this book is available from the Library
of Congress.

ISBN 978-0-7566-4171-9

DK books are available at special discounts when purchased
in bulk for sales promotions, premiums, fund-raising, or
educational use. For details, contact: DK Publishing Special
Markets, 375 Hudson Street, New York, New York 10014 or
SpecialSales@dk.com.

Color reproduction by MDP, Bath Altaimage, London
Printed and bound in Singapore by TWP

Discover more at **www.dk.com**

CONTENTS

Defining tantra

Tantra is an ancient Indian practice that is still relevant today. It celebrates the body and sexuality, teaching that the sexual act epitomizes your divine nature, and can lead to enlightenment. Tantric sex can bring vitality and intimacy to your relationship.

what is tantra?

Developed in India more than 5,000 years ago, tantra is a way of life that promotes the idea that sexuality, spirituality, and the emotions are all interconnected. Central to tantra is the belief that the human body should be celebrated and honored as a source of sensual pleasure as well as for its role in divine enlightenment. This is thought to occur at the perfect union of opposites, such as that of the male and female.

The tantric path teaches you that everything that occurs in life is a gift from which you can learn. The word tantra has many meanings, including "the way" and "transformation." As you move through this book, you will go on your own tantric journey. Your partner is a mirror to you, who journeys alongside you on the tantric experience.

achieving enlightenment through sex

First and foremost, tantra encourages you to enjoy sex fully, to cherish your body, and to make the most of every moment that you spend with your partner. Tantric sex is considered to be the fast track to enlightenment. When you reach orgasmic bliss during sex, tantra encourages you to bring full awareness to this state of being, and to stay in it for as long as possible. During this stage, you transcend into an experience of blissful awareness, free of desire, yet remaining fully conscious of what is happening. This state of mind is enlightenment.

space and retreat

The environment around you has an immense effect on your sensual and spiritual wellbeing. Tantra teaches you to create a sacred space in which to practice your meditations, whether at home or simply around yourself. Within this space you free

TANTRA TODAY

Tantra is very relevant for modern relationships. It encourages you to spend time together, to become more intimate, and to put aside the responsibilities and concerns of the world for a while. You embrace who you are today, right now. This is a radical departure from the quick-fix mentality of our society, where we're constantly trying to find fast ways to get better, richer, and happier. Tantra can make you feel more alive and more fulfilled in a simple, yet satisfying way.

In tantra we honor the divine in everyone and in everything. You will begin to see beauty in the world around you in places you never even knew existed. You begin to experience the simple things in life more deeply: a breath, a hug, and the beauty of nature. Your senses come alive, and you make time to indulge them.

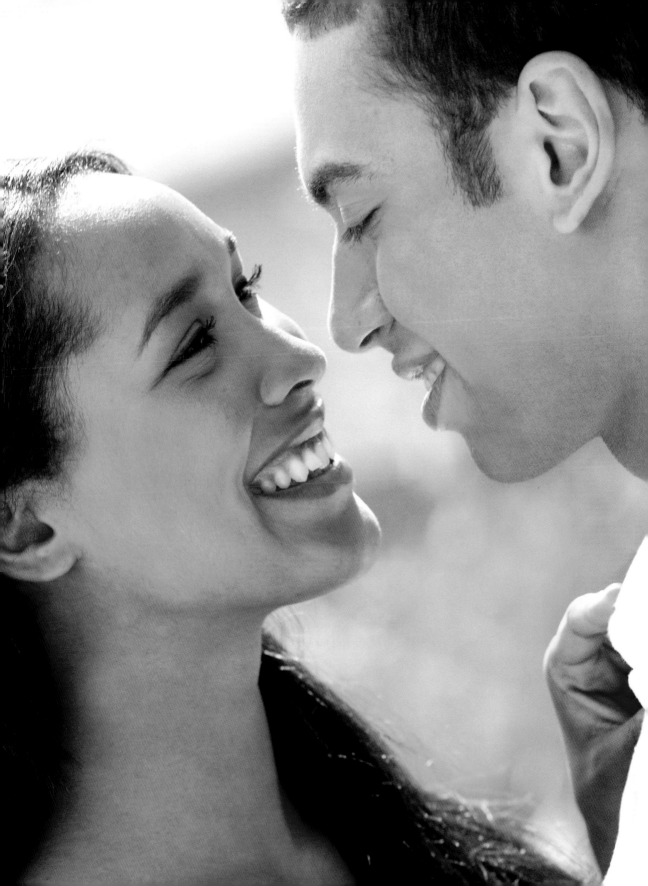

yourself from stress and worry, and focus on your tantric practice. Tantra also recognizes that it is important to get away, or retreat, from your usual space and routine, and to spend time devoted to yourself, your partner, and tantric meditation.

tantric meditation

Meditation is a way of observing the mind and focusing on being in the moment. Anything that takes you to a place of peace can be called a meditation, and in tantra we find meditation during sex, as well as in other ways. Many people tend to think of meditation as a quiet pastime, but tantric meditations can be very active, moving into still, meditative bliss after your bodies have exhausted themselves.

Try the meditations that feel right for you, make you feel sexy, and open your heart. You can dip in to tantra, choosing a meditation that appeals to you, or you can repeat one so that the experience can anchor itself deeply in your system. Some meditations take an evening, and others just ten minutes. Choose these if time is short, or if you are new to tantra.

the tantric lifestyle

Tantra teaches you to accept and enjoy your body the way it is, and also that it is important to look after your body, and to treat it as well as you can. Good food and exercise play an important role in tantra. When you eat well and look after your body, you can bring that energy to your meditations. Make healthy choices, and slow down, savor, and enjoy the food you eat. This is an important part of awakening your senses.

Practicing tantra is a good way to get more fit, and the healthier you are, the more you'll benefit from tantric meditations. Gentle but effective stretching such as Pilates, yoga, or Tai Chi helps you realize your body's strength and flexibility. Try to do something that gets your heart pumping regularly, and that makes you feel alive, whole, and vibrant.

Dance is an important part of tantra and features in some of the meditations that follow. It is a way of celebrating your body, your life, and your freedom of expression. You will notice that when you start to move, your mood will lift and your body will feel energized, alive, and very sexy. These feelings are the natural rewards of living a tantric lifestyle.

TYPES OF TANTRA

During its long history, there have been many strands of tantra. Below is a list of the main tantra lineages that have survived through the centuries, and that you may discover:

- Shiva tantra: This practice says yes to love, yes to life, and yes to sex. Every aspect of the human being and the whole of life is accepted and embraced.
- Tantra yoga: More male-oriented in its approach, saying yes to sex but no to love. Sex energy is used to launch the adept into spiritual consciousness, without the many emotional complications that can arise in love relationships.
- Tantric Buddhism: In Tibet, the meeting of Buddhism with the ancient Shamanistic Bonn religion created this unique fusion. Sex is allowed within a very precise framework, the goal of which is transcendence of the body.
- Taoist tantra: China has developed Taoist methods that use the vital energy accessed during the sex act to regenerate the body. A part of this teaching focuses on the retention of male ejaculation during orgasm as a way of staying young. It is a precise and technical methodology.
- Neotantra: A contemporary philosophy, based on a synergy of meditation and love. This highly relevant brand of tantra has caused a resurgence of tantric practice in the west over the past forty years, led mainly by the Indian tantric master, Osho.

This book presents an impartial view of tantra. It combines neo-tantra processes, more modern in flavor, and ancient rituals and meditations, to give you a chance to experience different facets of tantric sex.

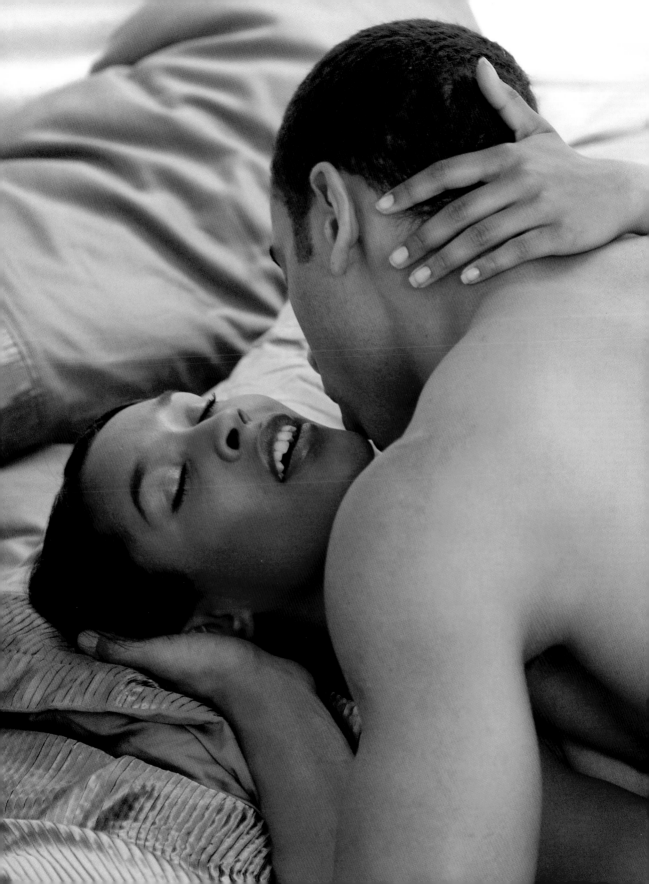

Tantric rituals

Simple ritual acts can bring richness and depth to life. Rituals are used in tantric meditation to calm the mind, and to focus your attention on your partner. A tantric ritual consists of a series of actions that will make lovemaking more intimate, meaningful, and pleasurable.

connecting through ritual

Sacred tantric rituals or ceremonies take you both into a deeper space of spiritual awareness and connection. They generate a feeling of reverence between lovers and are what create the distinction between sexual intercourse and tantric lovemaking. They also help you to focus on your partner, adopt a greater spiritual awareness, deepen your level of intimacy, and prepare you for the meditation and lovemaking to follow.

When you and your partner are new to tantra, the most important thing to bring to your tantric rituals is humour. Tantric time is playtime: a chance to awaken your senses and explore the wonders of being both human and spiritual. Don't worry if you feel nervous or self-conscious when you try these rituals for the first time. Laugh together to release tension, and focus on the sensual ritual steps, which will help you enter into meditation with a calm, focused spirit.

types of ritual

Rituals can be as simple or as complex as you like. The simple namaste ritual, for example, can be used on its own, or at the start and end of other ceremonies and meditations. The opening and closing ritual (overleaf) energizes you both before you start a meditation, and calms you at the end. The yab yum position (overleaf) is a wonderful ritual position that you can use to rest during lovemaking and at other times of intimacy.

As you start to bring more rituals into your everyday life you'll begin to notice how much they enhance your world. You become aware of each moment more clearly, and you make time to notice sensual detail and beauty around you. You may notice how your breathing calms and how your body relaxes.

RITUAL OBJECTS

To help focus your minds, you may like to include symbolic objects in your rituals. Tantra holds that certain objects can symbolize aspects of life—for example, a silver cup can represent the love union between two people. You may choose objects from nature to symbolize masculine and feminine, such as beautiful stones and shells (see page 50).

namaste ritual

Namaste is an ancient Sanskrit word that means "I bow down to the divine in you" or, "I honor the God or Goddess in you". This prayerful and highly potent greeting acknowledges the spiritual nature of your partner, and is often used to start a meditation. You can also use this ritual at the end of a meditation.

1 Kneel opposite one another and bring your hands together in prayer position (see right). Look softly into each other's eyes.

2 Close your eyes and bow down to each other, honoring the divine in your partner.

3 Come up with your hands still together. Look into each other's eyes again and say, "Namaste" (pronounced na-mas-tay).

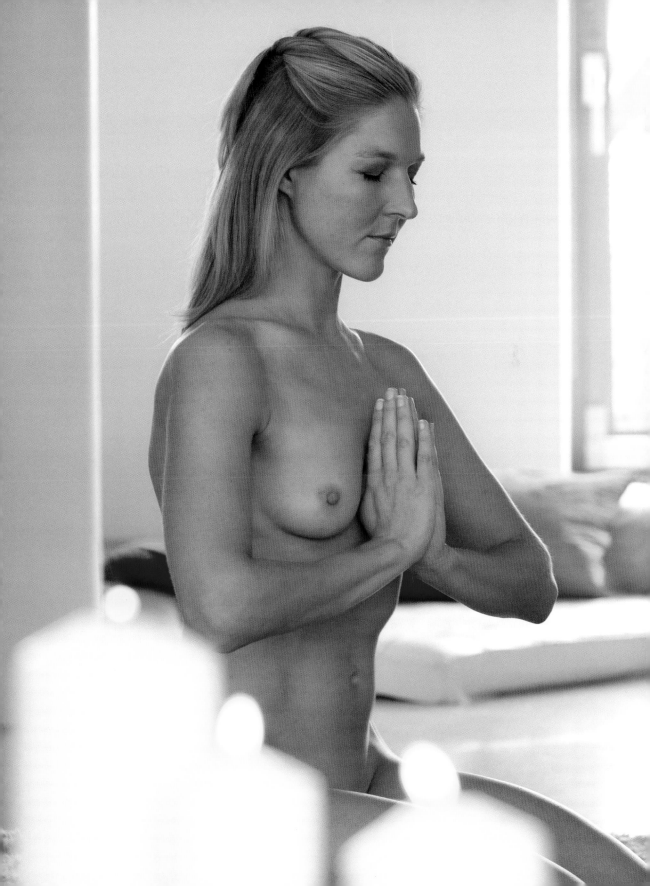

opening and closing ceremony

You can use this ritual to begin or end a meditation. If used at the start of a meditation, raise your arms upward in offering to the universal power that is greater than us, whether you know this as the Higher Source, Universal Wisdom, or God. As a closing ceremony, skip this step and focus on bowing down, paying homage to the love created between you.

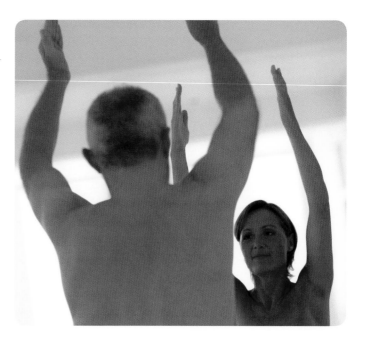

1 Sit opposite each other, on your knees, resting back on your heels.

2 Bring your hands to prayer position as you look softly into each other's eyes.

3 Raise your arms to the sky to offer your meditation to the universal power.

4 Bow down to the ground, and imagine pouring your ego down into the earth.

5 Raise yourselves up, and bring your hands together in prayer position. Look at each other and say "Namaste" to finish.

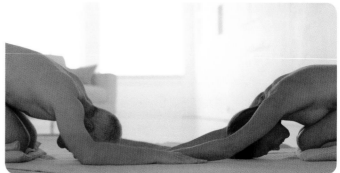

yab yum position

This position symbolizes the sacred union between masculine and feminine. You can embrace and rest in this position whenever you want to be intimate and hold each other. You can also use this position during lovemaking to cool the heat of passion yet keep your heart connection, especially if you want to delay orgasm or ejaculation.

1 The man sits cross-legged, in the lotus position. The woman sits comfortably on his crossed legs, and he holds her in his lap. She may like to sit on cushions to feel more at ease at first.

2 The woman wraps her legs around his back.

3 Place your foreheads together so the centers of your foreheads touch. This area is known as your "third eye" and is associated with psychic intuition and transcendence. Feel the deep, intimate connection between you, and enjoy the sense of feeling loved, safe, and powerfully connected.

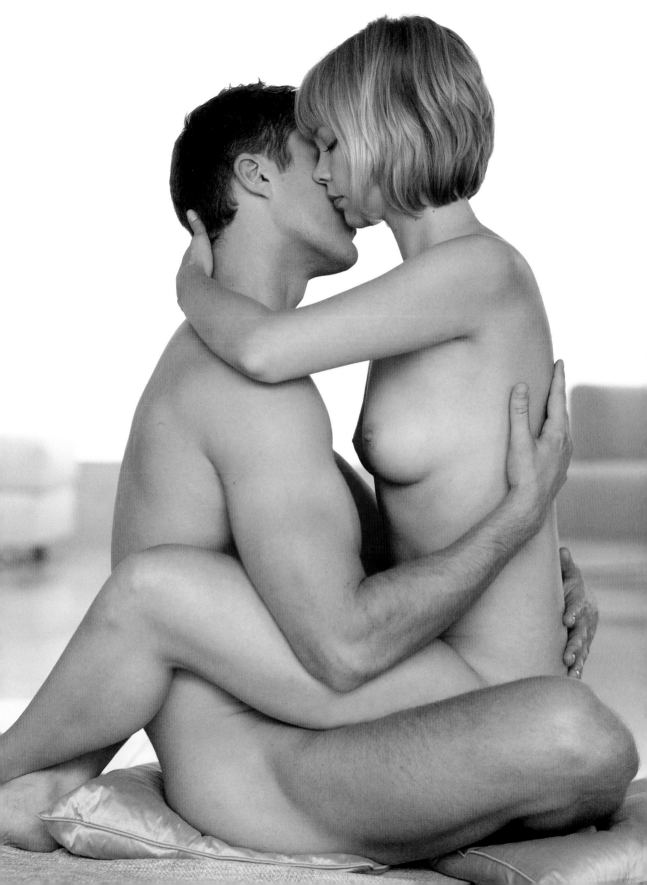

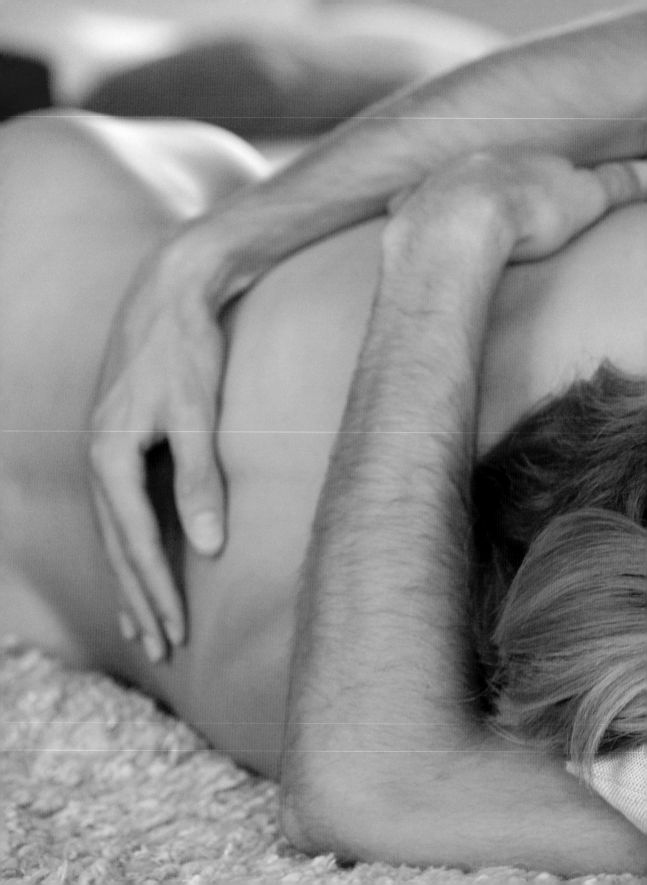

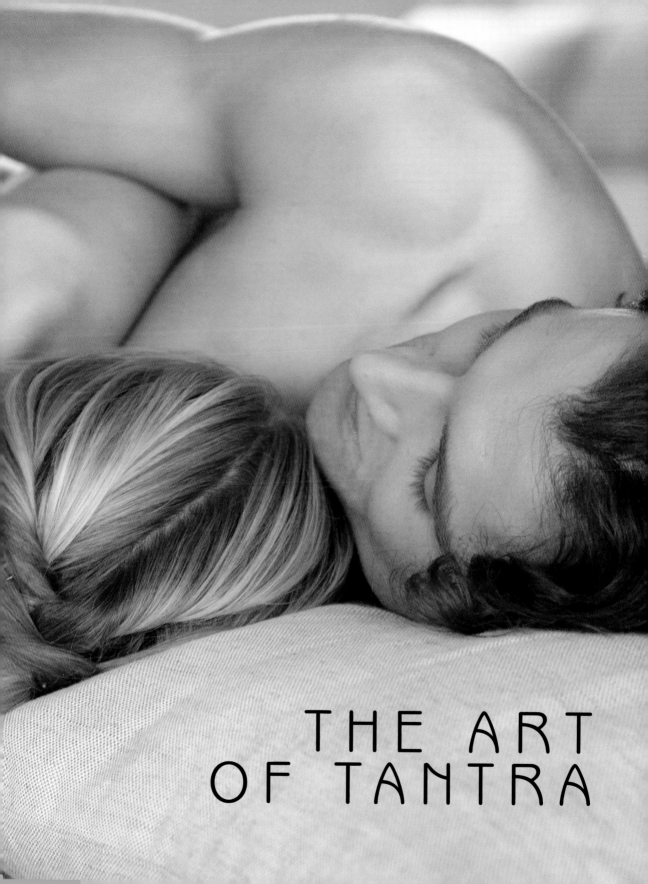

THE ART
OF TANTRA

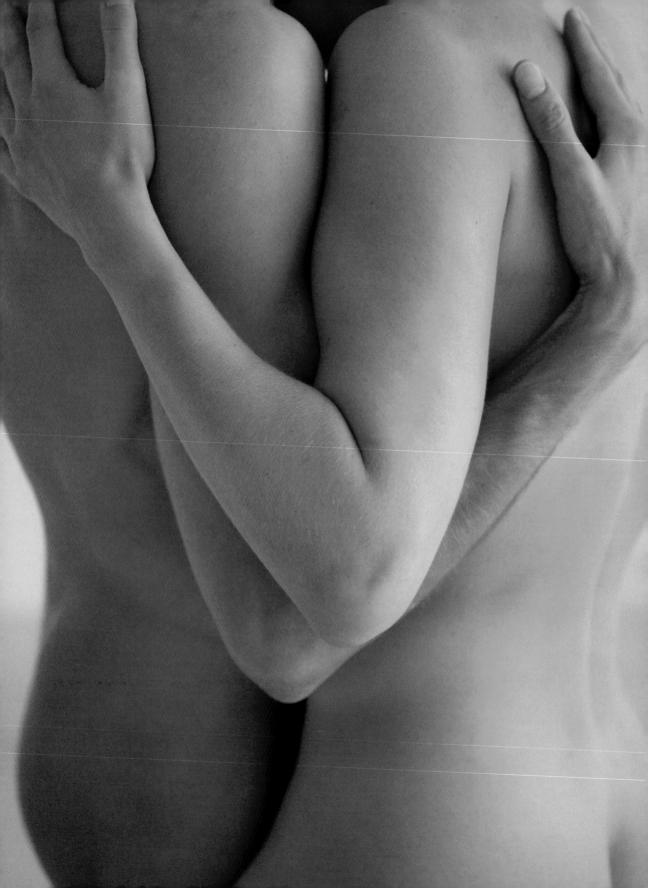

1

THE SACRED BODY

At the center of tantra is the sacred body. Tantric practice encourages the celebration of the physical, teaching you to nurture a relationship with your body patiently and kindly. As the hub of both spiritual and physical energy, the body is something to be cherished, cared for, and lovingly shared. Tantra awakens the body, and unleashes its beauty, strength, and sacred power.

Your body is a temple

Tantra celebrates the body as a physical representation of our divine nature, designed to be cherished as much as possible. When you embrace the erotic nature of your body, you are able to transcend the physical realm and access deep spiritual and sensual truths.

the body and tantra

Tantra invites you to bring full consciousness to your body and to access the orgasmic potential in everything you do. Understanding the sensations, feelings, and emotions experienced within your physical form is instrumental to feeling whole and fulfilled, and is ultimately the gateway to experiencing the divine energy of the universe. Your body is your temple, and during tantric meditations you and your partner will worship and honor each other, sharing pleasure, passion, and a deep awareness of your physical forms.

the erotic body

As you grow to be more in tune with your body, you will naturally become more aware of your own powerful eroticism. Tantric meditation encourages you and your partner to explore each other in new ways, using taste, scent, and sensual touch to come to a full understanding of the wonder of each other's bodies. You may be surprised at how this intimate exploration gives you greater intuition when it comes to your partner's emotional and spiritual needs. In tantra, body, mind, and spirit share a strong connection. This is one reason why tantric lovers spend so much time pleasuring and learning about the body. It is a constant source of discovery and enlightenment.

Make it a priority to set aside regular time to reflect on the beauty of your body–then revel in the pleasure that comes as a result. Tantric meditation gives you permission to worship the body often, and frees you to value physical pleasure in your relationship. As you move further along your tantric journey, your bodies will become temples that bring enlightenment, joy, and unending physical pleasure.

LINGAM AND YONI

In tantra we use Sanskrit words to describe the genitals, mainly because they are charming and evocative, as opposed to the rather clinical terminology used in the West. We refer throughout the book to the penis as *lingam* which means "wand of light" and the vagina as *yoni* which means "sacred space" or "cave of wonder".

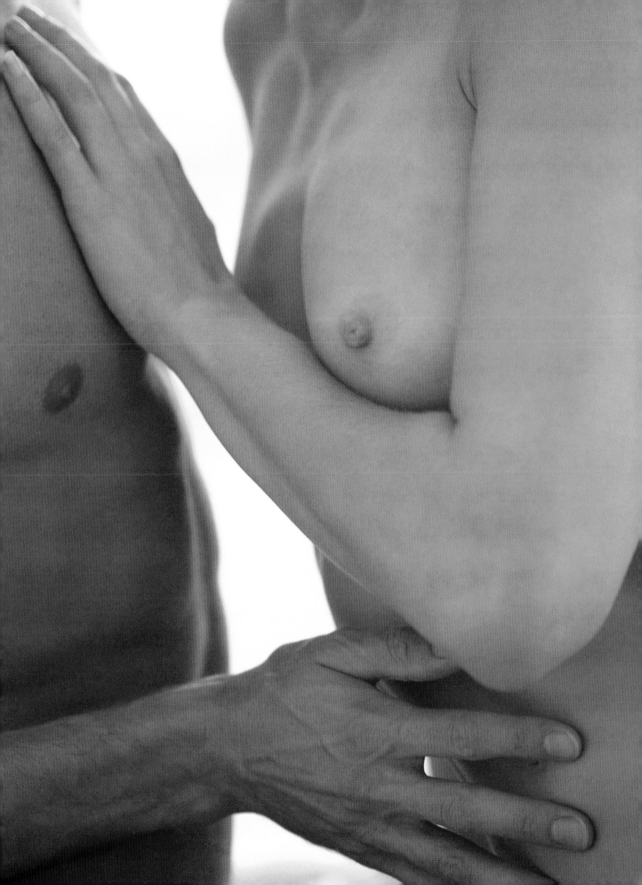

The seven chakras

Tantra teaches that you have seven chakras which are closely related to sexual energy and harmony. The intimacy and energy you feel when you are connected to your partner during meditation and lovemaking comes from having fully aligned, awakened chakras.

what is a chakra?

Chakras are energy vortexes, found both within your body and in your aura (the human energy sphere around your body). Tantra recognizes seven main chakras that lie within your body, positioned from the bottom of your pelvis to the top of your head. Each one is associated with qualities that are key to your personal wellbeing and your relationship with your partner.

The word chakra comes from the Sanskrit word *cakra,* which means *wheel* or *turning circle.* When your chakras are energized the energy literally spins. This can create a revolving door between your physical body and the mysteries of the universe, linking the spiritual and the sensual. As you spend more time in meditation, you will find that your chakras begin to open, creating a greater connection with your partner and a deep sense of physical and spiritual fulfilment.

how chakras affect you

When your chakras are open and energized you become more powerful and vibrant. You feel whole, alive, and intimately aware of yourself and the people around you. The central channel that runs from your pelvis up to your crown becomes a clear passageway through which energy can flow freely. This energizes every organ in your body, making you feel alert, positive, and passionate. You feel more connected to your sensuality, and more often in the mood for sex.

Most people have one or more blocked chakras from time to time, and this can be caused by tiredness, illness, or emotional concerns. Tantric meditations, especially those based on touch and massage, can help you to clear any energy restrictions in your chakras, and allow your full potential to flourish.

THE CHAKRA SYSTEM

Within the various schools of tantra there are different interpretations of the nature and role of each of the seven chakras. Here are the most common associations. You may also discover your own as you explore tantra.

 Seventh chakra
bliss, oneness

 Sixth chakra
psychic intuition, transcendence

 Fifth chakra
creativity, expression

 Fourth chakra
love, sacredness

 Third chakra
individual truth, egolessness

 Second chakra
emotions, feelings, sensuality

 Base or first chakra
sex, survival, lust

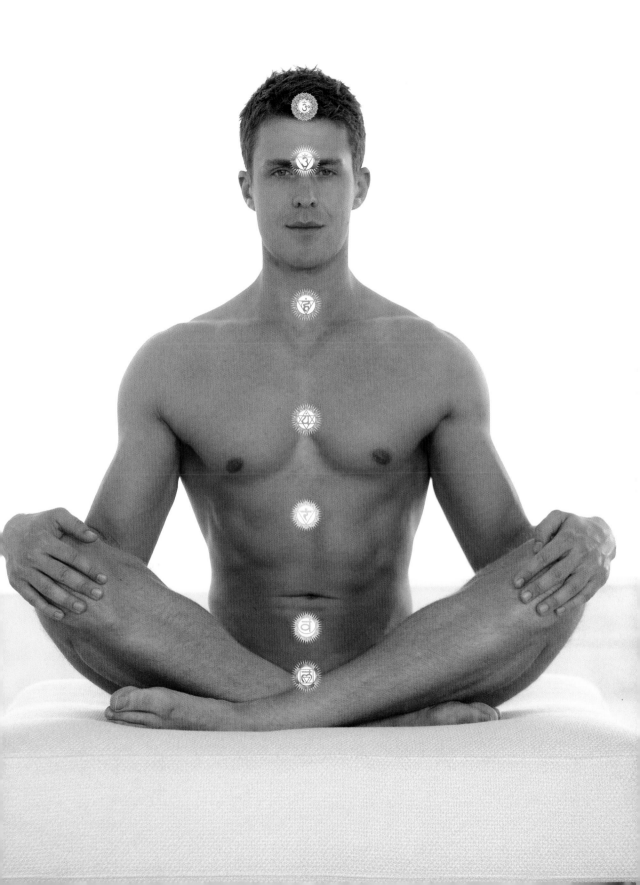

the relationship between male and female chakras

Men and women have the same chakras as each other, but they operate slightly differently. With the exception of the seventh chakra, the chakras complement and lock into each other, rather like magnets. For example, a woman's heart chakra is considered positive, and a man's is considered receptive. The sexual energy between a man and a woman is most powerful when these positive and negative charges unite.

The base chakra is where most of your sexual energy is focused. A man's sexual energy is transmitted out of his base chakra, through his lingam. A lingam's personality is stimulating and energizing and is considered a positive pole. A woman's base chakra is receptive. The yoni lies inside a woman's body, and the energetic personality of the yoni draws in and receives.

The chakra system plays a crucial role in the connection between two lovers. When a man and a woman are physically close there is a play of energy between their chakras, and especially between the first and second chakras that are related directly to sexuality. When your chakras are aligned, your senses are heightened and lovemaking can be electric.

If you feel you are not connecting as a couple, it may be because one or both of you has a chakra with a restricted energy flow. This is common. The movement of energy within you may change daily, but tantra can help to keep your chakras open.

connect your chakras

When your chakras are balanced and spinning together you can generate sexual electricity of the most potent kind. Even if you are already satisfied with your sex life, you can benefit from working with your chakras. You will find that communication becomes easier, that there is greater intimacy, and that you are more aware of when your partner wants tenderness or passion. You will also experience a heightened libido and greater orgasmic potential.

A number of methods can be used to balance and align the chakras and set them spinning. As you embark on your tantric journey, notice which meditations make you feel most alive, then include them in your chakra wellbeing program.

☙ Wake your male power

In some relationships men feel the need to hold back in some way, and may even be fearful of revealing too much of their male passion and energy. Tantra encourages you to express every aspect of your male power, and bring it to your partnership in a loving and considerate way.

A man's third chakra is the source of his strength and power. This chakra is located near the lower abdomen. Men often hold resistance in this area, especially if they have tried to conceal feelings, anger, or frustration over the years. If you hold your breath when feeling angry or frustrated, you can feel the tension in this area. The tension means that your third chakra is restricted, and that your emotional and sexual energy will also be restricted.

Giving attention to this area through massage can clear any energy restriction, and will help awaken your full masculine power. You can massage this area yourself, or your partner can do so. Use massage oil and rub the area in the hollow at the bottom of your rib cage using firm, circular movements. This can be done by itself, or as part of a full body massage.

massaging the second chakra

The second chakra is tied to emotion and sensuality. This massage is for the female partner to receive. Men will find their partner is more relaxed and open to intimacy after being stimulated in this way. Women will feel ready to receive their partner on a deeper level in whatever might be the next phase of lovemaking.

1 Namaste each other (see page 10).

2 Ask your partner if she'd like to lie down and be worshiped. She can be clothed or naked, however she feels comfortable.

3 Pour a little massage oil into your hands, then massage your partner's lower belly in a clockwise direction, slowly and methodically, using the flat of your hands, changing between hands with a gentle rhythm.

4 Encourage your partner to breathe into her belly while you massage. Remain conscious and present throughout. Notice her belly softening under your hands. Show your love and appreciation through your hands.

5 At the end of the massage, kiss her belly gently, with soft, delicate kisses all over, so that she feels loved and worshiped.

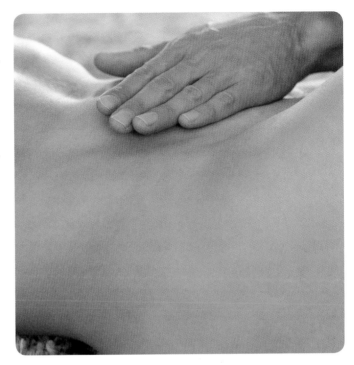

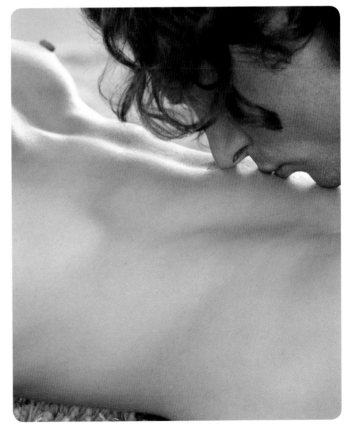

Tantra and self-image

Tantra teaches that a strong self-image comes from appreciating, enjoying, and pampering your body. When you do this, you will find that your chakras are opened more easily and that you are happier and more relaxed. This is the foundation of a healthy sex life.

honoring your body

Looking after yourself in a tantric way can be as simple as exercising regularly, receiving a calming massage, or enjoying healthy food. Find exercise that you enjoy, and make time for it. Walk in nature, stretch and strengthen your body with Pilates or yoga, or dance with your partner–anything that makes you feel happy, energized, and relaxed afterwards. Never feel guilty about making time for yourself; it is vital for a strong self-image and for the happiness of those around you.

self-esteem and sex

A satisfying sex life is one of the best ways to look after yourself. Sex can help you laugh, relax, and even sleep better. Notice how your body responds to making love: your senses are heightened, your pulse quickens, and you feel completely alive. You deserve to feel like this as often as possible. This starts with enjoying your body as an erotic, sensual entity.

Tantra heightens your senses and, as a result, changes how your body feels during sex. You will enjoy every sensation in a new way, thereby increasing your orgasmic potential. You can more easily imagine how your partner feels during sex. You feel positive and optimistic about life and your relationship, and experience a growing love and confidence. This positive energy then overflows into every aspect of your life, and makes others, including your partner, feel good around you.

When you bring this new perspective and energy to a sexual relationship, you are more likely to get what you want from your sex life. You will also find that you are even more sexy to your partner. A positive self-image and a well-loved body are equally necessary for a fulfilling, passionate, and adventurous sex life.

ᕬ rest and relaxation

Tantra teaches you to find bliss in any given moment, and this can be difficult if you are busy, stressed, or tired. Resting and relaxing provide a chance to breathe out and let go of pressure. When you feel rested and calm, you are more likely to want to move into intimacy and lovemaking with your partner, rather than dwell on the stresses of the day.

There are many things you can do each day to let your body and mind rest and relax. Make time each day for a short walk. Step out of the office at lunchtime or for a short afternoon break, take a stroll before your evening meal, and find a quiet, open space where you can relax, think, and meditate. You could take a bath or find a quiet space at home to sit alone for a few moments. Most of the time we don't realize how tightly wound we are until we spend time alone. Rest and your body will thank you for it.

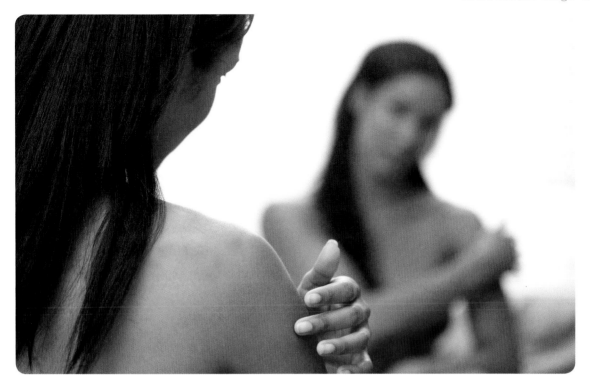

love and hate list

This is an eye-opening meditation to try if you are new to tantra. It will encourage you to identify the areas that you like about yourself, and to begin to appreciate each part of your body as uniquely yours. Do this exercise alone first, then try it with your partner. It is a sensual way to express all the things you love about each other.

1 Draw two columns on a piece of paper with one column headed "love" and one headed "hate."

2 Stand naked or simply dressed in front of a mirror. Look at yourself and write a list of all the things you dislike or hate about yourself. You may write a part of your body, or a personality trait. Be honest and write what comes first.

3 In the other column write a list of everything you like or love about yourself. Compare the length of each list.

4 Put on some sad music and for a few minutes imagine that you are one of the features on your hate list. Dance and emote fully all the aspects of that feature, for example, if you don't like your legs, touch your legs, caress them, and over-emphasize feeling fat or wobbly, or whatever you think.

5 Now change the music to something positive and uplifting. Choose a feature from your love list. Touch and caress that part of your body, and focus on the texture or color, or whatever it is you like about your feature. If you love your full breasts, stroke them, shake them, and exaggerate their presence as you dance.

6 After dancing three or four features from each list, look at your lists again and see if there are any features that you can move from the hate to the love side of the page.

7 Do this exercise every day, for as long as it takes to move all the features from the hate column to the love column. It is completely feasible for you to be able to empty the hate side and fill the love side. Over time your feelings will change, and you will feel kinder toward yourself.

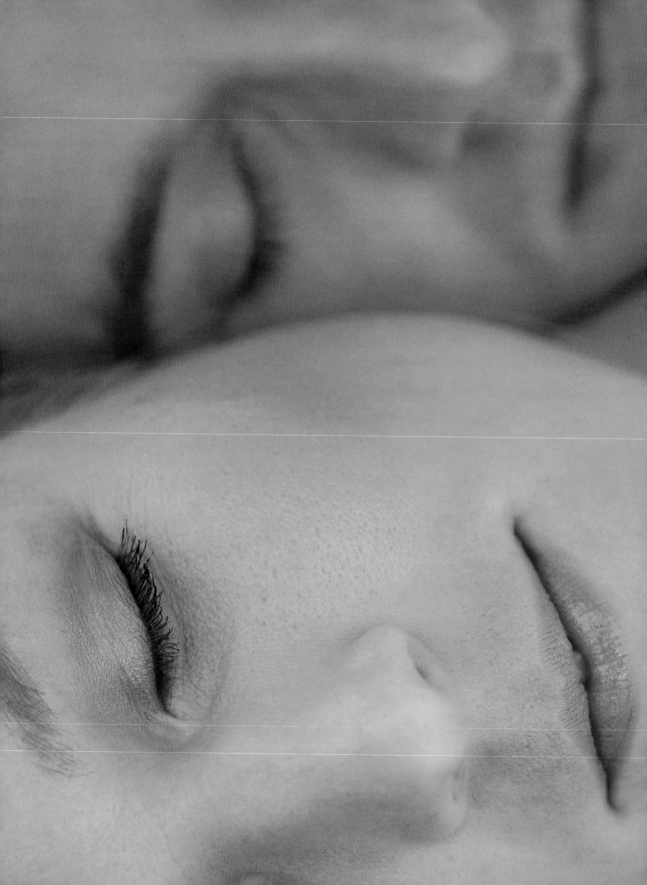

2
THE SACRED
RELATIONSHIP

Tantra invites you to look at your relationship with consideration and warmth. By devoting time, energy, and passion to the most important person in your life, you will experience immense joy, adventure, and intimacy. Your sexual union is a sacred and divine act, and can help you to access cosmic bliss together.

Shiva and Shakti

The divine tantric relationship is based on the model of Shiva and Shakti, believed to be the first couple to practice tantra. Their passion, wisdom, and deep connection were fostered through creative meditation, intimate communication, and passionate lovemaking.

the masters of tantra

Nearly 5,000 years ago, Shiva and Shakti originated and practiced the first tantric meditations, which were recorded as the *Vigyan Bhairav Tantra*, a series of 112 sutras. The sutras are still practised today, and provide steps for building intimacy, deepening relaxation and self-awareness, and embracing new techniques in lovemaking. Many are included in this book.

Little has been written about Shiva and Shakti's human lives, although there are various theories as to who they were before becoming immortalized as tantric gods. All of these theories suggest that Shiva and Shakti were a curious and creative couple, who shared a vibrant sex life and a thirst for spiritual knowledge. Their relationship was defined by mutual respect, shared creativity, and deep passion.

the divine masculine and feminine

Shiva and Shakti represent the different qualities of the divine male and female. Embracing your true nature as a divine man or woman has a powerful effect on your relationship and your sex life. Merging gender-specific strengths—such as Shiva's creativity and Shakti's compassion—makes for an irresistible sexual and emotional connection between two people.

Start by noticing how these qualities play out in your relationship, and how you can use them to enhance the time you spend in meditation together. Tantric practice can give you space to express elements of your nature that may be hidden in other areas of your life, such as at work. In tantra, you can put aside the role you play during the day. Over time, you may feel able to bring your full Shiva or Shakti personality to all areas of your life.

YOUR DIVINE NATURE

Shiva's qualities are:	Shakti's qualities are:
strong	receptive
rational	loving
vibrant	mercurial
playful	giving
powerful	maternal
active	caring
creative	heart-led
wise	compassionate

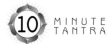

10 MINUTE TANTRA

SEEING THE DIVINE

This meditation encourages you to see the divine in your partner. You can use this way of seeing each other in later meditations.

1 Sit opposite each other comfortably.
2 Look softly into your partner's eyes. Breathe slowly and deeply. Let any irritations and upsets that may have accumulated in the day fall away. Resist the temptation to talk to each other.
3 See if you can recognize the divine in your partner. Look deep into the ocean of your partner's soul and meet beyond your personalities, responsibilities, and mind-games. Aim to connect with your partner's spirit-flame, the energy within them.
4 Remain lost in the gaze for at least five minutes. Move and stretch to finish.

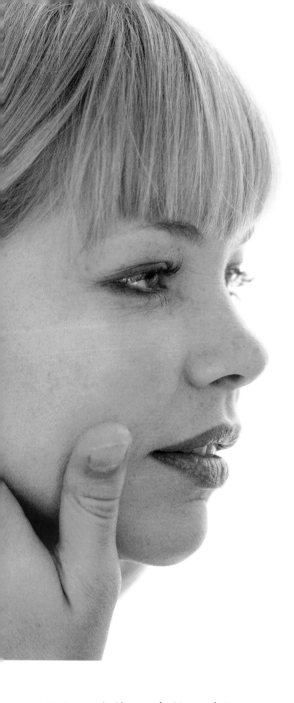
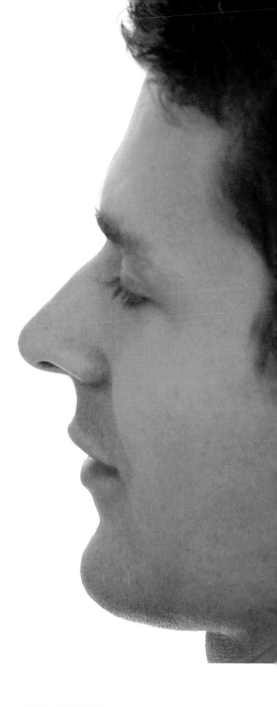

an exquisite relationship

When Shiva and Shakti met in sexual union, they created an exquisite friction and great erotic energy. This frisson and fusion of energy is what creates life and brings blissful, orgasmic fulfilment. As you begin your tantric journey, learn to welcome and embrace the differences between you and your partner, and enjoy the friction that you create together.

ROLE REVERSAL

Women can also embody the attributes that are typical of Shiva, and vice-versa. Tantra recognizes that we hold the potential of all aspects of humanity inside of us, both male and female, and we should embrace that.

The union of opposites

The tantric path to bliss is through the conscious union and merging of masculine and feminine forces. Focus on bringing the strongest elements of your characters to tantric meditation and you will discover the same lasting passion that Shiva and Shakti shared.

communicating with your partner

Because male and female natures are so different, the communication between you and your partner is very important. Tantra invites you to exchange ideas with each other through talk, touch, play, and lovemaking, just as Shiva and Shakti did. Set aside time to tell your partner about your feelings and desires, and to bask in the spiritual and sensual enlightenment that comes as a result.

rediscovering your partner

If you want to awaken and ignite, it is important to accept and embrace each other's differences. It is your differences that create the sexual spark of energy and excitement that can propel you toward orgasmic bliss. Women, admire your partner for his strength and masculinity; men, adore your partner for her sensual nature. It is both thrilling and daunting to open up new avenues of expression in a love relationship, especially when you are in a defined relationship pattern, but the risk is one worth taking. When you make the choice to add this risk and vulnerability to your relationship, you will reap the benefits in a number of different ways.

Most couples long for that honeymoon phase where they enjoyed each other's differences, and things were new and exciting. Imagine what might happen if you put aside an hour or two every week to connect again with your partner. If you have lost sight of what made you sexy and appealing to each other in the first place, spend time away from cares and responsibilities, focusing on different types of touch and communication. Let tantra give you a path to rediscover–and add to–the characteristics that you once found so attractive.

YIN AND YANG

The ancient Chinese teachings of Taoism defines the masculine principle as "yang" and the feminine principle as "yin." The opposing qualities of yin and yang are present throughout the universe, and are responsible for friction, change, and energy. Yin and yang have equal power, and together they enrich and energize the other, bringing fulfillment.

YIN	YANG
Femaleness	Maleness
Moon	Sun
Completion	Creation
Cold	Heat
Darkness	Light
Material forms	Heaven
Submission	Dominance

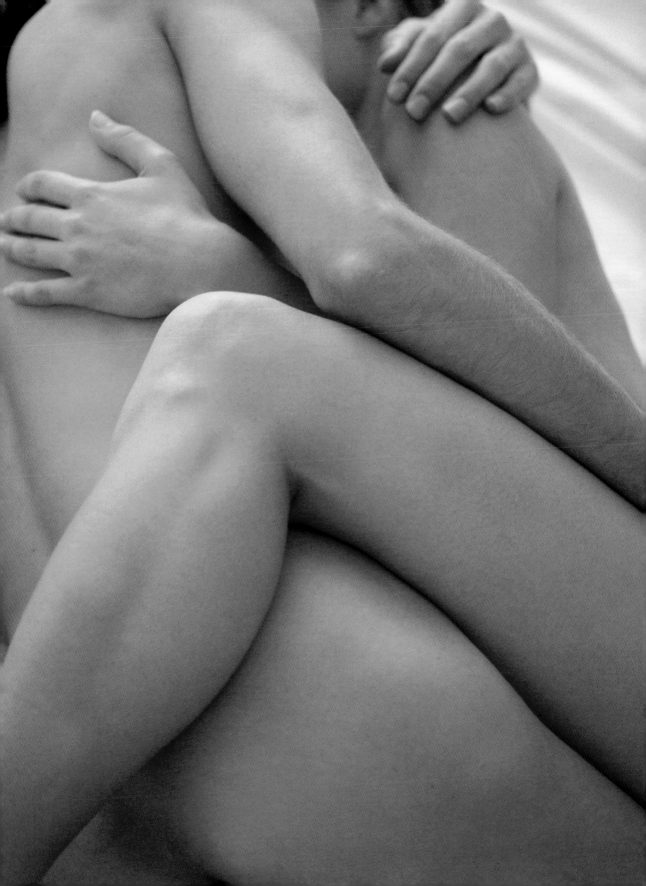

yin yang touch

This meditation can help both of you to communicate and teach each other, without any words, the kind of touch you enjoy. The roles of giver and receiver become deliberately confused, creating the tantric experience that giving and receiving are entwined and are equally pleasurable. Change position throughout to stay comfortable.

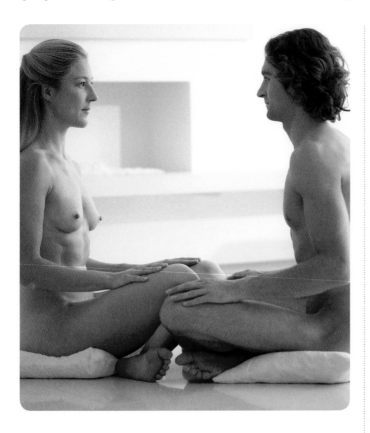

☌ Touch awareness

When you are the partner being touched, try and feel the exact quality of the touch your partner is giving you. Notice the intent and message in the touch, if it is gentle and tender or erotic and playful. Learn to keep your awareness on the touch and respond with your body, and don't filter it through your mind. Let your body respond. This tantric touching will begin to feel like making love.

1 Sit opposite each other, and namaste your partner (see page 10).

2 Decide who will be the initiator, yang, who determines what happens, and who will be the follower, yin, who puts their own wishes aside for the time they are in this role.

3 Yang begins to touch yin in the way in which he or she would like to be touched. Yin gives back the touch she is receiving. It might take a few moments to respond in the same way, but soon your reaction times will speed up, so that you touch simultaneously.

4 Yang should keep the touches slow and flowing so Yin can follow easily. Try not to make sudden movements, as this would mean Yin would need to focus more intently.

5 Think about the touch you desire, and touch your partner in this way. Emphasize any features that are missing in the response, for example, if your partner is going too fast, make very slow movements. If you need to speak, don't criticize, simply ask calmly and kindly.

6 After about seven minutes, change over. Continue taking turns until each of you has had three turns. You can follow this meditation with lovemaking if you both desire.

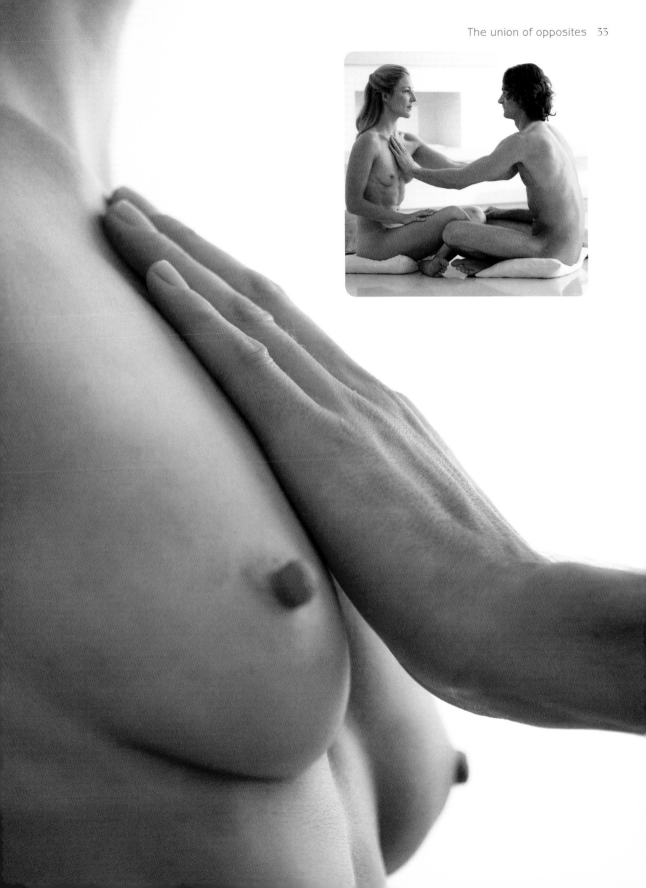

Your tantric relationship

As you and your partner continue on your tantric journey, you'll find that the connection between you sizzles in new ways. Continually nourish your relationship with time spent in meditation and intimate ritual, and watch your relationship flourish in trust and love.

tantra, you, and your partner

As you explore tantra, remember that the relationship between you and your partner is sacred. Your love is a gift, to be treated with reverence and respect. Be gentle with each other as you navigate new territory. Try new things, and listen to your partner to find out what he or she does and does not enjoy.

One thing you'll notice during your tantric journey is that you will both begin to slow down, and to spend time getting to know each other again. The methods in tantric meditations are simple, yet the transformative effects can be life-changing and can bring new energy to a long-term or even fading romance. Even if you feel happy in your relationship, tantra can help you discover new ways to enjoy your time together.

Listen to your partner as you try new meditations, and discover what works for you both as an emotional and sexual partnership. Find rituals that you both enjoy and learn from. Notice and acknowledge your different desires, emotions, and feelings, and allow these to be fully present during sex, and in other parts of your relationship.

the love body

Your relationship actually has three components–you, your partner, and the love body of the relationship itself. Think of the love between you as a separate entity, with its own force and energy. This love body needs to be nurtured with attention and time. Spending time together, enjoying your bodies, connecting in meditation, and being kind to each other will help your love body to flourish. Tantra helps you reframe your ideas about love, sex, and the importance of your relationship, allowing you to move to new levels of understanding and intimacy.

ଽ Tantra for singles

If you are single or your partner isn't ready to step onto the path of tantra, you can still practice meditations alone, reaping great benefits. Tantra can help to raise your self-confidence, and encourage you to enjoy life to the full. The positive energy that comes from time spent in meditation will bring benefits to all your relationships.

If you would like to find a tantric partner, there are several ways you can do so. One of the best is to go on a singles tantra course. These focus on connecting, sharing, intimacy, and personal growth; you are never expected to have sex. You could also join a tantric dating agency, which will put you in touch with other members who are actively studying and practicing tantra.

how to start on a tantric journey

Throughout your tantric journey, you will discover pieces of an ultimate truth—one that comes from your heart and not just your head, and that will bring us more happiness, freedom, and love. If you feel that it is natural for romance to diminish over time, or that you know everything about each other already, start to replace these old relationship myths with positive ideas such as:

• Love is infinitely expansive
• I can grow and learn through a love relationship
• Everything that occurs in our relationship is a gift

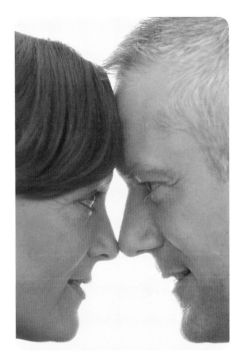

These will help open your mind to new ways of thinking about your relationship. Start doing simple meditations by yourself and with your partner. If your partner has hesitations about joining you, keep extending the invitation, without too much pressure. Tantra cannot be forced, and it is important that you both feel comfortable with beginning this journey together.

You may also choose to go on a workshop, alone or with your partner. This can be a valuable way to learn about tantra, though it is important to remember that there are as many different styles of tantra as there are styles of yoga (for a summary, see page 6). Keep investigating courses and teachers until you find one that appeals to you and meets your needs.

rising in love

Tantra replaces the traditional idea of "falling in love" with that of "rising in love." This reflects a creative and positive intention, and allows you to truly open your hearts, minds, and bodies to each other. You will become more intuitive toward your partner, and will be able to anticipate his or her desires. During meditation and lovemaking, you will experience an enhanced pleasure that is only possible with perfect intimacy.

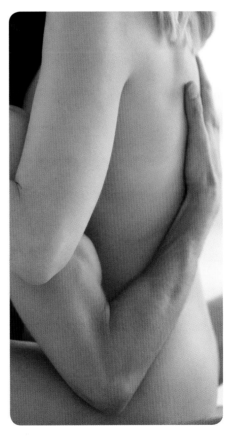

Rising in love will help you look at your partner with new eyes, and will add a sense of adventure to your relationship. Be creative with each other, and build up your love relationship with frequent meditation, talk, touch, and lovemaking. As you try new things in tantra, you will experience your partner in new ways. You will also discover different aspects of yourself that you can bring to your partner. Look for new discoveries in your tantric relationship, and rise in love together.

nurture your love body

This meditation can help both partners get used to the idea of sharing a tantric experience, especially if one or both of you are new to tantra. It is an excellent way to think about all the good aspects of your relationship, and also to raise any concerns you may have as you start on your tantric journey together.

1　Namaste each other (see page 10), then sit or kneel comfortably next to each other.

2　Place an object (try a cushion or chair) in front of you. This will represent the love body of your relationship. Each place a flower in front of you.

3　Take turns speaking to your love body directly, talking about your experiences within the relationship, your partner, and any concerns or issues that may have arisen lately. Talk about your partner in the third person. For example, "He makes me laugh" or "I think he is keeping something from me." Include what's pleasing you and what's bothering you. Take five minutes each, alternating in your sharing. Each time you speak, allow yourself to go a little bit deeper and take some risks in your sharing. Don't interrupt your partner when he or she is talking.

4　When you reach the end of the sharing, each pick up your flower and imagine pouring your ego into it. Visualize all of your mind chatter and all of your limiting beliefs leaving your mind and pouring into the petals of the flower. Take a couple of minutes for this, then lay your flowers next to each other before your love body. Feel the physical lightness resulting from letting go of your concerns.

5　Bow down and ask for wisdom or guidance from your love body. If you are quiet and drop all expectations, an answer should form in your mind. Trust what comes, no matter how silly it sounds to you.

6　Sit up and share the advice or insight with your partner by whispering it into his or her ear.

7　Hug, then namaste each other to finish.

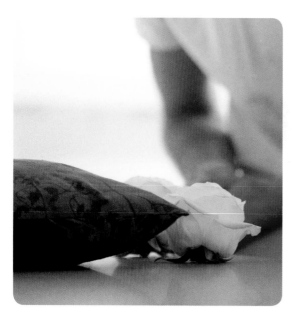
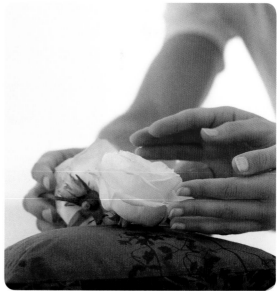

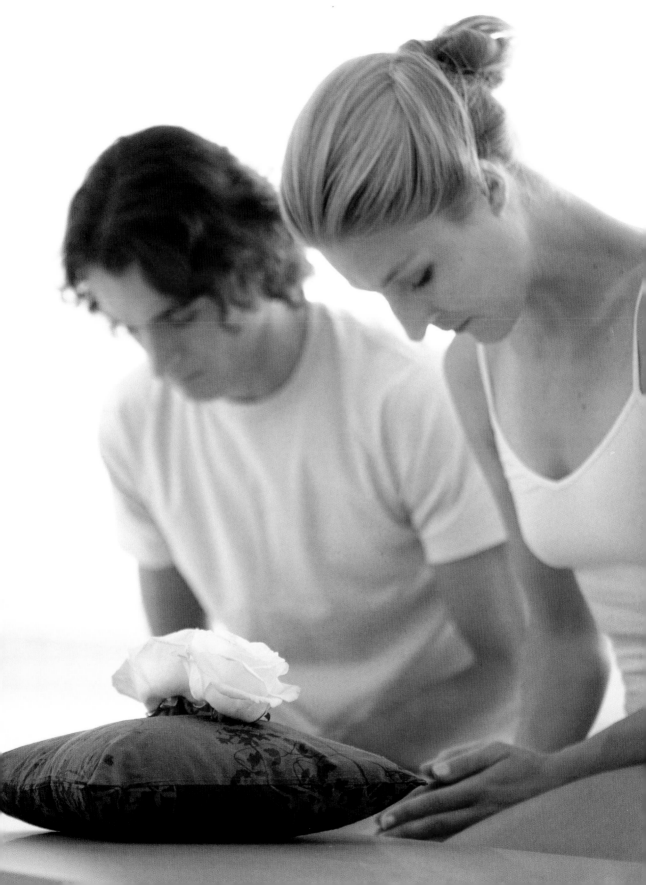

Emotional release

Releasing any emotional issues from your past is an important part of your tantric journey, and allows you to move forward in your relationship. Identify, express, and embrace your emotions, then allow them to fully flavor your sexual relationship.

embracing your emotions

Learning to work with and embrace your emotions as opposed to resisting them is an important stage in liberating yourself so that you and your partner are ready to go forward on your tantric journey together. If you suppress your natural feelings and desires, you may gradually diminish your capacity to feel strongly about anything, including love and sexual feeling.

expressing anger

Anger, for example, is a natural human emotion that many people tend to feel uncomfortable discussing and expressing. There is a belief that anger is something bad, and should be ignored, but it is a vital part of being human. Many people are afraid that if they access and express their anger, they may lose control or do something they regret. Tantric meditations can teach you to express and release anger in a non-aggressive way. You are most healthy and alive when you recognize and express all of your emotions, whatever they may be.

emotions and your sex life

If you make an effort to forge a healthier relationship with your emotions and learn how to express them, you will become a more open and honest lover. Clearing the obstacles to a fully alive and enriching relationship can take willingness and humility from both partners, and tantric meditations can give you the structure to do this in a safe, supported way.

Tell your partner when you feel angry or tired, but also remember to tell them when you feel happy and full of vitality. Bring this to your sex life together: notice when your partner is tired and wants gentle attention, but respond with vigor when he or she seems energized and ready for passion.

YOUR EMOTIONAL BODY

Your body speaks volumes about your emotional state and where you are in your life. In Chinese medicine there is a map of how organs and emotions fit together. If you have a chronic health issue, look first to see if you're having problems with the emotion relating to that area of the body. These may be the emotions to give special attention to during your emotional release work.

- Genitals, kidney, and bladder: Fear and trust
- Liver and gall bladder: Anger and spontaneity
- Lungs and large intestine: Sorrow and inspiration
- Heart and small intestine: Joy and love

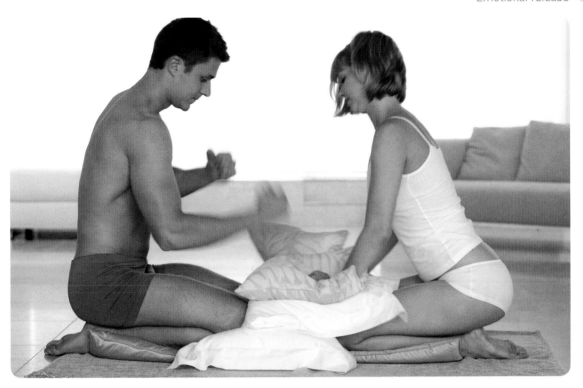

pillow beating

You can do this emotional release meditation on your own or alongside your partner. It can help you to release any buried feelings, especially those of anger, sadness, and despair, in a responsible, safe way. Pillow beating literally shakes and wakes up any suppressed life force energy.

1 Place a large pile of pillows or cushions in front of you, and a beautiful flower next to you. Sit on your knees, using another cushion if that is more comfortable. Namaste your partner if you are working together (see page 10).

2 Put on loud, aggressive music. Come up on to your knees and raise your hands, clasping them together above your head. Bring your hands down onto the pillows with passion, shouting "No!" loudly. Keep going, using all your force and energy.

3 Shout "no" as many times as you like, then voice sentences that express your feelings. Dump your feelings into the pillows. Scream at your partner, if you like, but keep hitting the pillows. The music should be loud enough so that you can't hear clearly what each other says. Feel empowered, knowing that you are choosing your own words. Continue for five minutes, and stop together.

4 Sit quietly for five minutes, letting your breath slow down. Close your eyes and let whatever needs to happen, happen. If you feel like crying, allow the tears to come, but move into silence and stillness as soon as possible.

5 Take the flower into your hands together, and imagine pouring each of your egos into it. Bow down, placing your flower next to the pillows. Visualize this as an imaginary altar of love, which also represents your emotional healing.

6 Hug, and then lie together for at least 10 minutes. Be sensitive to each other, but don't discuss what happened. There is no need to try and fix anything; allow everything to be as it is. Rest in your partner's presence and enjoy the intimacy that follows such an emotional outpouring. If you are working alone, lie quietly, enjoying a sense of peace and love.

The sacred union

A union is the merging of two or more elements to create a harmonious whole. Tantric meditation fosters a sacred union of body, mind, and soul. This leads to a better understanding of your partner—and also to the deepest possible physical pleasure.

connecting during sex

Tantric sexual union is different from most sexual union, in that it encourages you to fully revel in every aspect of your union, including the sacred and spiritual. Tantric meditations are the best way to experience and understand this. When you try a meditation you are encouraged to focus on one or more elements of your union, such as a particular sense, or to rise and rest in valleys and peaks of desire. Rather than being focused purely on ejaculation or orgasm, you learn to enjoy every moment, every look, and every touch. Each moment of your union has the power to transport you toward spiritual bliss. You take your time so as to prolong the blissful experience, and to build and heighten your pleasure.

your divine partner

You also honor your partner during tantric sex by getting to know him or her on a deeper, more profound level. This helps you to discover more about your lover, allowing him or her to grow in love and sexual fulfillment. The meditations in this book are practical methods to help bring greater levels of desire to your sexual relationship, along with more sacred meaning.

If you remain in contact with the wonder of existence during lovemaking, then the highest "rising" in love is possible. This experience is the ultimate aim of tantra, and it is what brings sex into a spiritual realm. Be in touch with the divine in your partner at all times, if you can. You can achieve this by dropping judgements and moving beyond his or her surface personality. Look into the deepest nature of your partner's being, touch his or her body with love and reverence, and learn to soar together, powered by your blissful connection.

speaking your desire

This sharing of desires can be about anything, including sex and sexual fantasies. This exercise will help you and your lover understand each other better through expressing your uncensored desires in the moment. During the meditation you will find that your mind will spill out its wishes and demands until they have been exhausted, creating a relaxed sense of space and freedom.

1 Namaste each other (see page 10).

2 One partner starts by saying, "I want…" followed by the first thing that comes into his or her mind. Let your desire be expressed as a stream of consciousness. Don't censor your thoughts. Let even crazy thoughts arise and express them. Don't be shy. You might say "I want…"and then there will be nothing but silence, and this is fine, too.

3 The other partner then declares his or her desires, "I want…"

4 Share like this, taking turns, for half an hour, until you have exhausted your thoughts.

5 Namaste again, to finish.

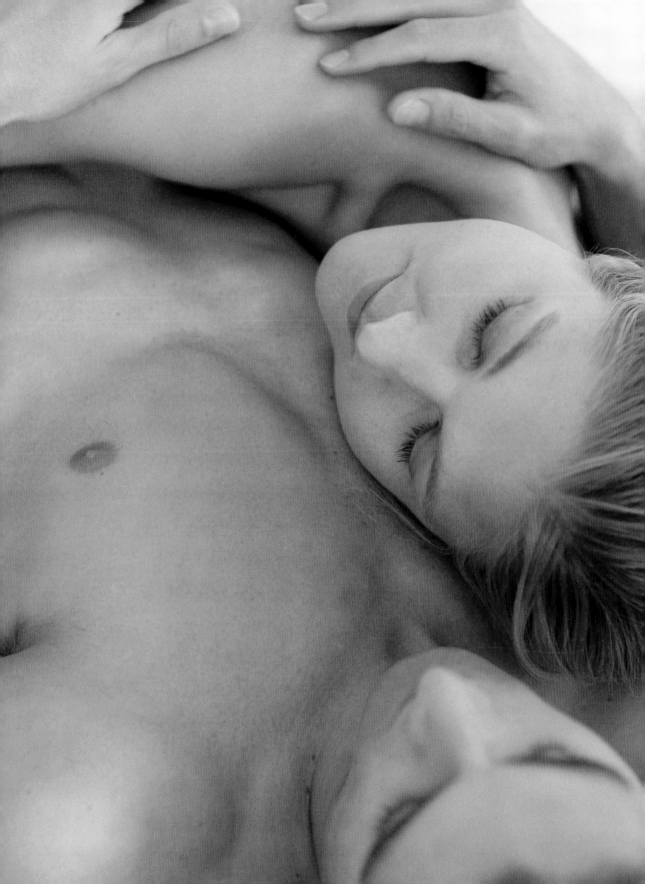

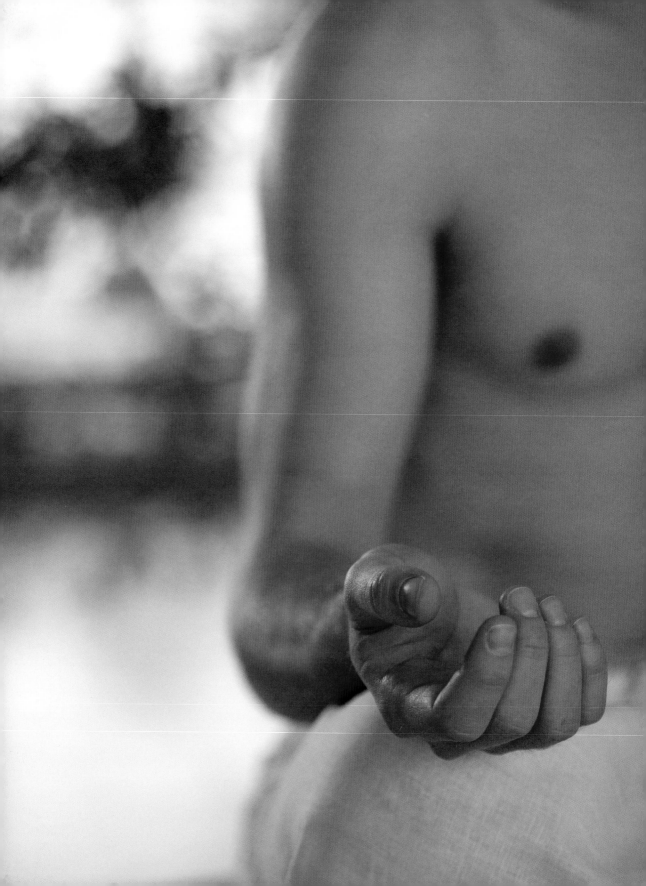

3

THE SACRED
SPACE

A relaxing haven away from the rest of the world is the ideal space to practice your tantric meditations. Whether an entire room or a quiet corner, a designated sacred space can help transport your mind and body away from your everyday life. Calm colors, scents, and soft, luxurious fabrics soothe the mind and body, creating the perfect place for intimate, escapist lovemaking.

Creating a tantric space

As you practice tantra, your senses will become more attuned to color, scent, and atmosphere. Clutter can distract you both, so a clean, calm environment will enhance the time you spend with your partner, and help to create a sense of ceremony.

why you need a sacred space

Although it's not necessary to wait until the conditions and environment are perfect in order to practice tantra, a quiet, beautiful space can help you to create an atmosphere conducive to meditation. By bringing attention to the details you can create a magical, sacred space away from the rest of the world. When you are both in your space, it is easier to focus on your partner, and to bring each other pleasure and joy.

The ideal scenario would be for you to dedicate an entire room to your tantric practice, but a corner of a room or your bedroom can work very well. With a thoughtful choice of colors, fabrics, and ritual objects, you will be able to create a haven of serenity to which you can escape and enjoy your time together. The visual ambience of your space is worth investing in. If your space looks and feels welcoming when you step inside, you will want to spend time there.

If you don't have room in your home to create a separate tantric space, transform what is already there by using items that are only for your meditations. A special bedspread, beautiful candles, a yantra (see page 51), or a wall hanging depicting tantric worship can help to transform your room.

space and sensuality

Tantric ritual and meditation bring a sense of sacredness to lovemaking. The environment in which you engage with your partner should have an aura of serenity and harmony. This helps to relax both of you, and bring your minds to the moment. Surround yourselves with beautiful things, and you will feel sensual and enlivened.

initiating your space

Before you start to use your sacred space create an auspicious beginning by performing a ritual. You can invent your own ceremony by following your intuition, or you can use the ceremony below:

1 Sit opposite each other comfortably and namaste your partner (see page 10).

2 Close your eyes and chant the universal sound "Om" three times (see page 98).

3 Sit quietly and feel your body expanding into the space around you.

4 Open your eyes and look into the face of your beloved. Say together: "We offer our meditations to higher consciousness. May our space be blessed."

5 Raise your arms above you. Feel energy filling your body and entering the space. Bow down to the ground, with your arms forward.

6 Namaste to finish.

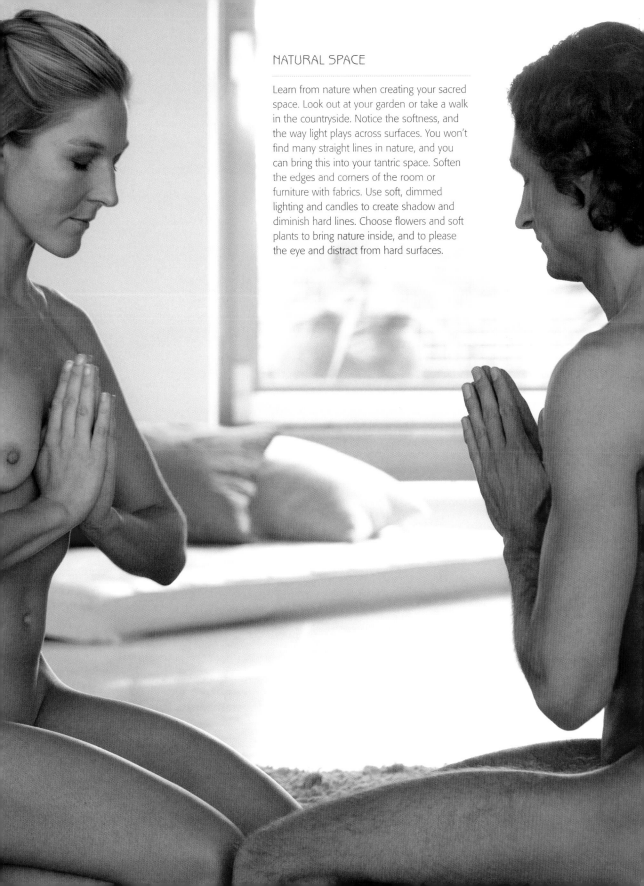

NATURAL SPACE

Learn from nature when creating your sacred space. Look out at your garden or take a walk in the countryside. Notice the softness, and the way light plays across surfaces. You won't find many straight lines in nature, and you can bring this into your tantric space. Soften the edges and corners of the room or furniture with fabrics. Use soft, dimmed lighting and candles to create shadow and diminish hard lines. Choose flowers and soft plants to bring nature inside, and to please the eye and distract from hard surfaces.

choosing colors

Color is energy, carried to us on waves of light. Like notes of music, each shade carries a different vibration. We are beings made of energy, so we resonate with color in a very personal way, depending on our own unique, vibrational quality.

Because of this, color can be an important part of your tantric experience. Bring colors into your sacred space that appeal to you. Traditional tantric colors are rich, inviting, and evocative– for example, red, burgundy, orange, terracotta, purple, saffron, and ocher. These colors stimulate the chakras and awaken the senses. They also charge the space with energy, creating a spiritually uplifting atmosphere in which to practice tantra.

You can sense what colors feel right for your own personal meditation space. Close your eyes and imagine a color: the first one that comes into your mind is generally your guiding color. This is the color that brings out the best in you, making you feel alive and sensual. Think of other colors and shades that enhance your feeling of wellbeing and mood, then integrate them into your space with paints, fabrics, and flowers.

sensual lighting

Candles have a magical quality that brings a beautiful softness to tantric meditation. Candlelight is the visual equivalent of a feather stroke, and is soothing and gentle. It is easier to relax in a room lit by candles: self-consciousness evaporates more naturally; your eyes soften so that you see with grace and sensitivity; and your heart expands in the muted light. It gives a very different feel to a tantric meditation to practice it in broad daylight, when you tend to be more analytical, and are alert to every sensation and emotion that is exchanged.

Be creative with the way you light your space but don't feel you need to have it a certain way in order to jump in to a tantric meditation. Tantra is a constant experiment, and can bring enlightenment in many different environments.

scents

According to ancient tantric teachings, smell is the sense that most ignites sexual energy and enhances sexual pleasure. Incense and perfumed oils were used in ancient tantric

COLOR AND THE ELEMENTS

Here are some examples of how colors are associated with certain elements. Notice how you respond to certain colors, and bring the ones that appeal in to your sacred space:

Red
passion, strength, energy, fire, love, sex, excitement, heat

Yellow
sunlight, joy, happiness, earth, optimism, energy

Orange
happiness, energy, balance, heat, fire, enthusiasm, playfulness

Purple
creative, meditative, unites the wisdom of blue and the love of red

White
purity, enlightenment, peace, tranquility, calm, harmony

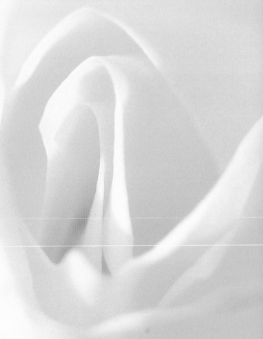

ceremonies to create a sacred ambience, and to enhance spiritual and sexual rituals. You can find references to sandalwood, musk, aloe, and camphor in the tantric scriptures.

Ideally, the scents you use in your sacred space should be natural. Essential oils distilled from natural sources, such as flowers, herbs, trees, and fruits are known to enhance sexual experiences. They can help to transform your mood, create an atmosphere conducive to transcendental lovemaking, and help you gain access to your spiritual self.

It is worth investing in an aromatherapy oil diffuser for your tantric practice. You can keep it burning with tea lights for hours, and it's easy to add aromatic essential oils at different moments in your love play. These scents can be chosen to match the peaks and valleys of your passion.

THE COLOR WHITE

White contains all of the colors. If you hold a glass or crystal prism up to pure white light it splits into separate colors, including each of the seven chakra colors. When your chakras are vibrating in harmony, this effect happens in reverse: their colors merge to make the beautifully pure white light of enlightenment.

No wonder white is seen by many as the color of purity, peace, and tranquility. White sheets and white rooms make us feel peaceful because we respond instinctively to white's simple message beckoning us toward the state of union that each of us craves. Incorporate white elements into your space to invoke a calming sense of rest.

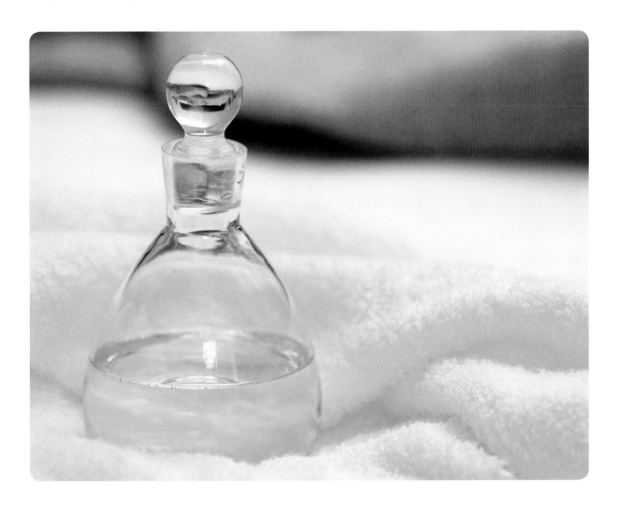

fabrics

You and your partner want to have the sense of being nurtured and pampered in a womb-like space. It is important that your room makes you feel secure enough that you'll feel disposed to removing your clothes and relaxing in a state of complete surrender, so choose items in fabrics that are soft and sensual to the touch. Velvets, silks, cashmere, and brushed cotton reflect opulence and luxury. Avoid harsh, man-made materials such as nylon and polyester. When choosing fabric, it is worth spending a little extra money to gain the quality that will add luxurious softness to your tantric sanctuary.

Place pillows and cushions of different sizes on the bed and around the room for reclining on. Choose ones that are large enough to kneel or sit on comfortably, consider which colors appeal to you both, and bring sensual luxury to mind. Softer pillows can make longer meditation times more enjoyable.

A large, soft rug such as lambskin is ideal for lying on together. Choose at least two gorgeous, soft blankets to include in your space, so they are to hand to cover up during meditations if you feel chilly, instead of having to put clothes back on. Consider purchasing two lambs' wool, mohair, or cashmere blankets that feel sensual, warm, and indulgent. Choose these with your partner, selecting materials that feel best for you both.

Invest in high-quality bed linen that you both like. Cotton with a high thread count of over 400 means that your bed will feel soft and luxurious when you lie naked on it. Make your bed feel like a real escape from the world by draping generous amounts of sheer fabric such as white or colored muslin over your bed to create a canopy. When filled with gorgeous bed linen and specially chosen cushions, this bed chamber will become a womb-like environment where you can fully relax and indulge yourselves away from the world.

CHOOSING AROMAS

A seductive blend of aromatherapy oils that is ideal for tantric lovemaking contains neroli absolute, rose, and jasmine. You can also create your own blend, depending on what aromas you or your partner are drawn to, and the atmosphere you would like to evoke:

Sandalwood
evokes sensuality and calms the mind

Frankincense and cedar wood
bring serenity and peace

Benzoin, black pepper, and ginger
bring warmth to the heart and body

Clary sage
can bring a state of euphoria

Jasmine absolute
enhances male sexuality, relieves sexual tensions

Rose absolute
a feminine scent, good for love, healing, and seduction

Neroli absolute
soothes anxieties, boosts virility and fertility

❦ Tantric music

Calming or stimulating, music helps to create a mood and transport the mind. Find music that you both like and bring it into your sacred space. Keep a music player in easy reach. You'll find suggestions for music in the Resources section (see page 186). Vary what you listen to during your meditations, to change your mood and the way you respond to the meditation.

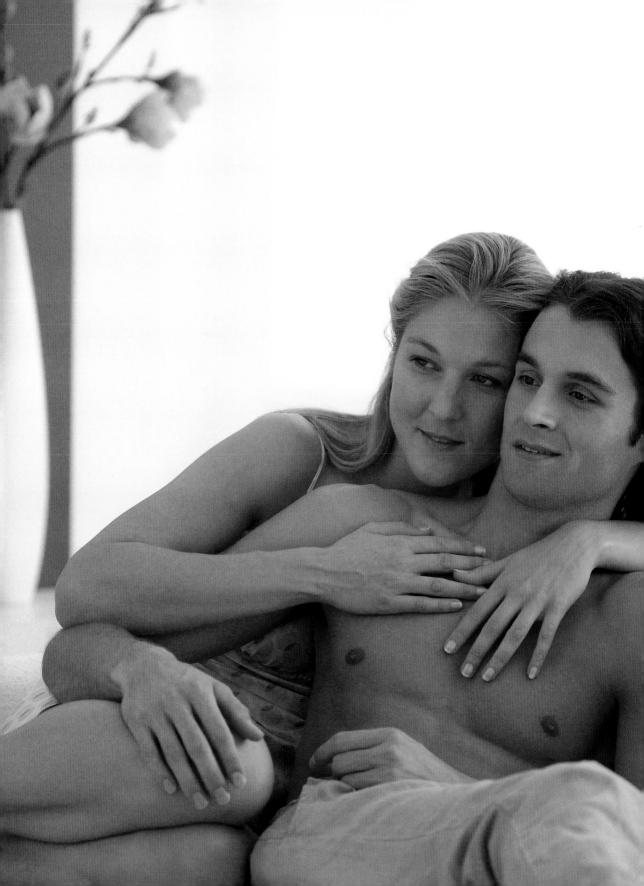

Ritual objects

Having ritual objects in your sacred space creates a potent feeling of love and sensuality that can enhance your tantric experience. Any item that is special to you can be used as a ritual object. You may also like to include traditional tantric symbolic choices.

personal objects

Objects can have special significance for the person using them in relation to their own unique spiritual path. You may feel drawn toward simple, natural shapes, or more exotic, explicit representations. Choose what feels appealing to you and your partner, and change items as you feel like it. Make an effort to keep your tantric space free of any objects that don't have special meaning relating to your tantric practice.

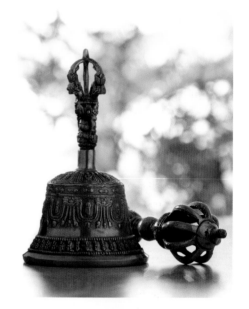

natural objects

Nature is filled with objects that can enhance your meditations. Reminding us of our connection with nature, many objects show characteristics of the masculine and feminine. These beautifully suggestive objects help keep us in touch with our own sensual and erotic nature. Look for shells, rocks, and pieces of wood shaped into forms symbolizing male and female aspects. The conch shell, for example, is a glorious representation of the yoni, with its hollow form and pale pink color, corresponding to the vagina and labia. A rock or piece of driftwood may have characteristics reminiscent of the lingam.

tantric objects

Throughout the centuries of tantric meditation, some objects have come to symbolize spiritual concepts. You can use them during meditations, or to bring new energy to your sacred space.

Shiva lingam

Egg-shaped stones found in Indian rivers, formed naturally by the river's current, are known as shiva lingams (see right), and are said to have one of the highest-frequency vibration rates of all the stones on earth. They are gathered on one day each year and are hand-polished to give them a smooth surface. The shape

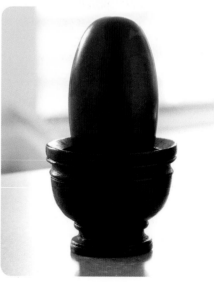

of the stone represents male energy and knowledge, and the markings, which differ greatly from stone to stone, represent female energy and wisdom. Together, the two elements signify the merging and balancing of male and female energy. In India these magnificent stones are regarded as sacred and holy.

Vajra and bell

In Hindu and Tibetan tantra, the vajra (see opposite) represents the male principle, and the bell represents the feminine principle. The Hindu deity Vajrasattva is often pictured holding the vajra in the right hand and the bell in the left. This symbolizes the tantric union of opposites that leads to enlightenment.

Yantras

A yantra is a form of mandala (see page 108). Yantras are beautiful pieces of art, made up of geometric and archetypal shapes and patterns. Yantras are created to embody the energetic blueprint of the universe, and meditating upon a yantra is said to invoke a higher state of consciousness. There are many yantras to choose from, including painted or woven pieces. If you find a yantra that speaks to you, try displaying it in your sacred space as a focus for meditation, or as the starting point for an altar.

Ritual trays

In ancient tantric practices, ritual offerings formed the basis of tantric worship. To bring this in to your tantric play, choose any tray that appeals to your senses. Then prepare your tray with love before a tantric meditation, with fruit, incense, flowers, and wine or juice. You and your partner can take turns feeding each other from your tray in recognition of your divine spirits, and to help each other to relax and unwind. This is a wonderful way to start or end a meditation.

Tantric cup

You may like to purchase a special goblet to symbolize your love union. Choose any design that appeals to you both. This cup will be used for sharing wine or juice during tantric meditations. Many tantric meditations are specially designed to help you focus on your senses of taste and smell. Display the cup on your altar and keep it only for use during tantric meditations. This way, your tantric cup will become charged with your passion, and whenever you sip from it you can imagine that you are drinking from the eternal source of your love.

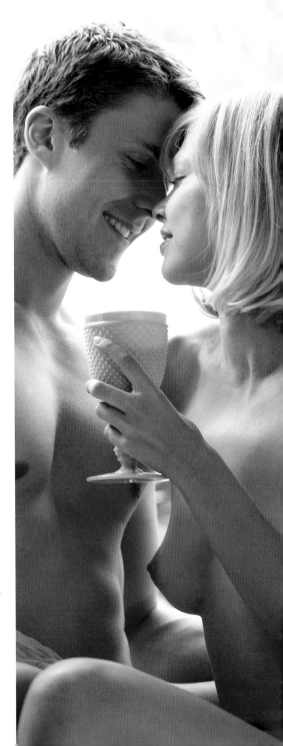

Altars

An altar serves as a beautiful, symbolic representation of your inner world, and the ideas and thoughts that are important to you. Your tantric altar can be a special place for you to meditate, honor your relationship, and give focus when you enter your sacred space.

the purpose of altars

An altar can represent your divinely spiritual nature–it is the outer expression of your heart. Your altar can also be a point of focus within your tantric space, for use before, during, or after your tantric meditations. You may find that spending time meditating in front of your altar alone or together will awaken your senses and increase your sexual energy as you leave the worries of the day behind you and focus on your sacred union.

When you create an altar with your partner, you are performing a sensual act of love together. Each time you return to your altar you will remember this process, and the meaning behind each chosen object, and again deepen your intimacy.

Altars radiate their own energy that blesses and sanctifies you, your partner, and your home. Just passing by and looking in the direction of your altar can bring you back to your essential nature, reminding you of who you really are, and encouraging you to be aware of the moment of now.

creating a personal altar

Your tantric altar can be as simple or as monumental as you like, and can be constructed in your own home or outside, in your garden or in nature. There is no design plan for the perfect altar, and it should spring up organically from the depths of your imagination. Use your intuition to locate objects that are meaningful to you and represent your own unique journey in this life, just as you did when incorporating objects into your sacred space. A traditional tantric altar would include items that represent the four elements of nature–fire, water, earth, and air, so you may choose to include those (see above), although you can also add more modern elements if they appeal to you.

৯ Designing your altar

One way to start to build a powerful altar is to incorporate the four primary elements—fire, water, earth, and air:

- Fire can be represented by a candle.
- Water can be represented by a bowl of water in which you might place some flowers or float some candles.
- Earth can be represented by a rock, shell, or crystal.
- Air can be represented with incense.

Add items that have a particular meaning for you: a photograph of the two of you together; a piece of jewelry that holds specific significance; or a favorite flower in a small vase. You may include sensual tantric objects that you can touch and caress, such as a shiva lingam or conch shell, or a statue of Shiva and Shakti in the yab yum position.

Find things that resonate with you and your partner, and perhaps inspire you to think about lovemaking. Is there something that reminds you of a special night away together, or an object that you exchanged early in your relationship that makes you smile when you look at it? Your altar is the place to keep it.

EARLY ALTARS

Archaeologists have discovered remnants of altars in the dwellings of many ancient civilizations. The simplest of objects have been used to create an altar, including animal skulls, which have been found decorated with flowers and precious stones.

blessing your altar

When you have placed your chosen items on your altar, you can inaugurate it with this simple meditation. You can write your own blessing or use the words suggested. As you meditate in front of your altar, think about the items you have chosen and what they mean to you and your partner.

1 Light a candle and sit or kneel comfortably in front of your altar, either alone or with your partner.

2 Bring your hands together. Bow your head slightly, look up, and say: "I declare this altar a sacred place of devotion and prayer. It symbolizes the perfect balance of inner and outer polarities. With an open heart I offer the truth of who I am."

3 Sit with your eyes closed and in silence for at least 10 minutes, focusing on your breath, and on the peaceful intimacy that radiates from your altar.

4 After the meditation, place your hands in prayer position and bow down again, allowing a refreshed sense of gratitude to pervade your whole being.

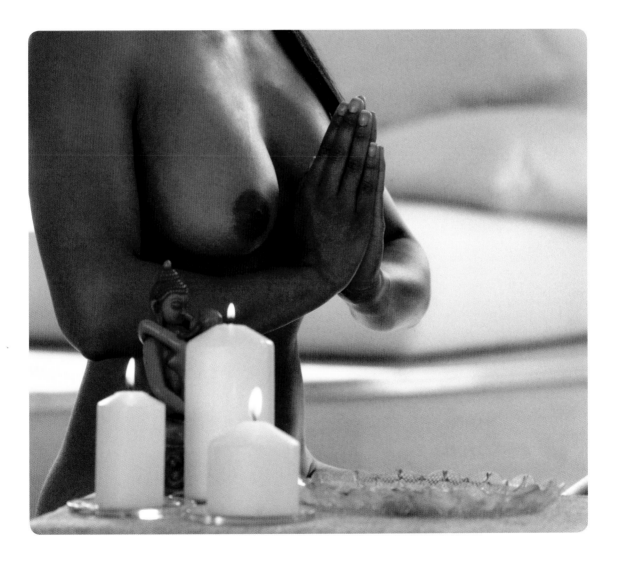

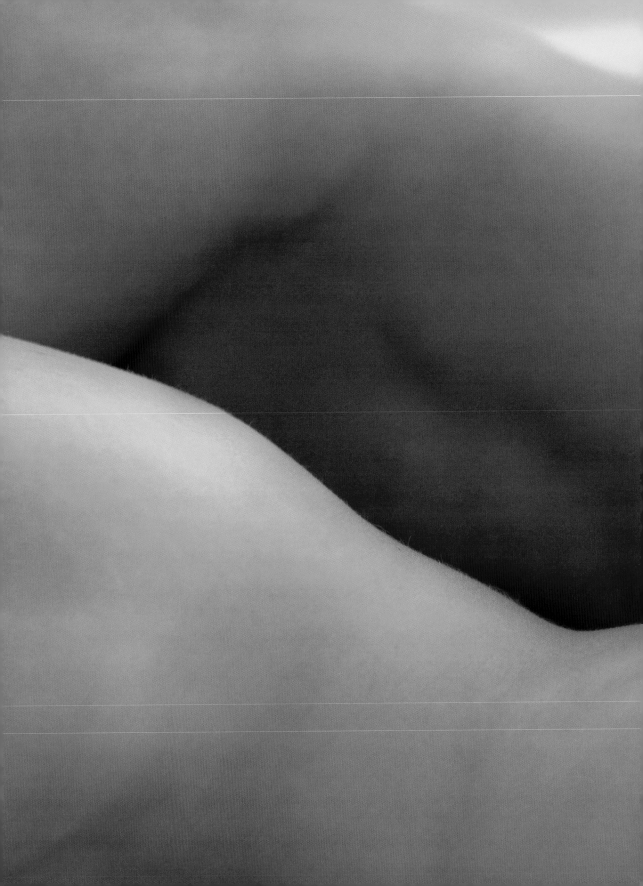

THE TANTRIC
CONNECTION

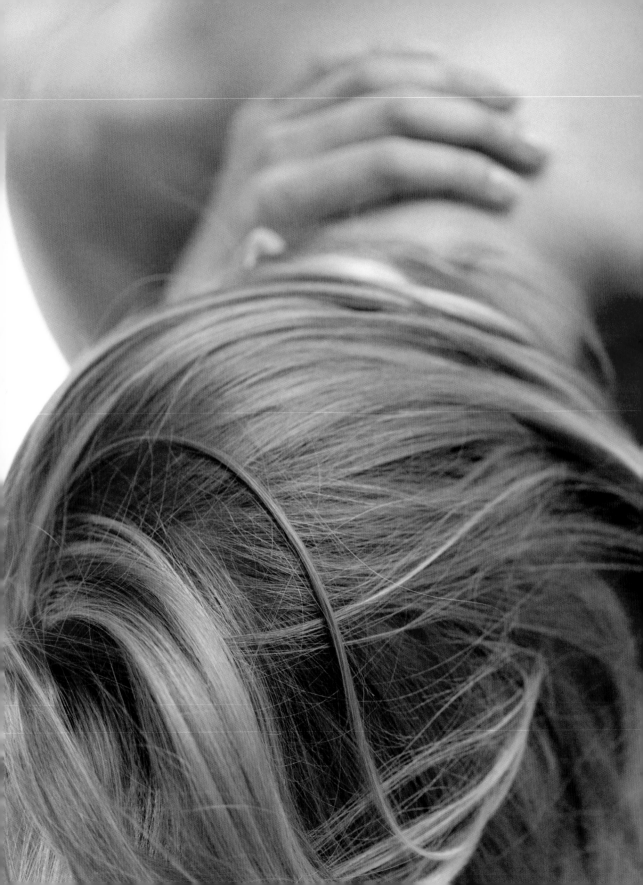

4

ENGAGING WITH YOURSELF

Only when you are bursting at the seams with vitality and happiness can you truly give yourself to another. A healthy self image is the foundation for your fulfilling, passionate sex life. When you are overflowing with health, positivity, and confidence you can embark on a truly rewarding tantric journey.

Self-exploration

In order to be in touch with your body's full capacity for pleasure, it is important to free yourself mentally and emotionally. Tantra encourages you to spend time exploring your mind and body, and thinking about your desires. These are the first steps toward a satisfying sex life.

exploring mind and body

Developing your mind is as important to tantra as developing your body, since your mind plays a leading role in all sensual experience. To understand on a deep level that you are the master of your own universe, creating your life as you move through it, it's vital to spend time in thought, unencumbered by the pressure of having to interact with, or take care of others. It is also important to get to know your body, how it works and feels, and to give it the physical attention that it needs. Create time and space for the things that relax your mind and arouse your body, whether it is a long shower or vigorous exercise.

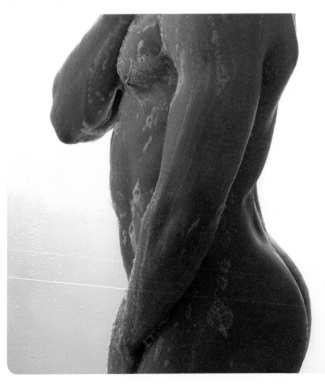

writing a stream of consciousness

Try this exercise to help you explore your mind and to get to know yourself. Let your "mind-chatter" tumble out.

1 Take a pad of paper and write down the thoughts that come into your mind, in a steady stream of consciousness for five minutes. It might not make sense but let the words flow in quick succession, without censoring.

2 Read the words out loud to yourself. Notice what goes on inside your head, and if your thoughts are positive or negative. Don't try to force them into any kind of order—just let them be as they are.

3 When you've read your mind-chatter, tear the paper up, throw it away, and sit in silence for five minutes. Let your thoughts float away and notice how clear-headed you feel.

GIFTS TO YOURSELF

Each day, give yourself at least one treat to show that you value and appreciate yourself. This could be a walk in the woods, a long bath, or extra time alone with your partner. Remember every day that you are worth it!

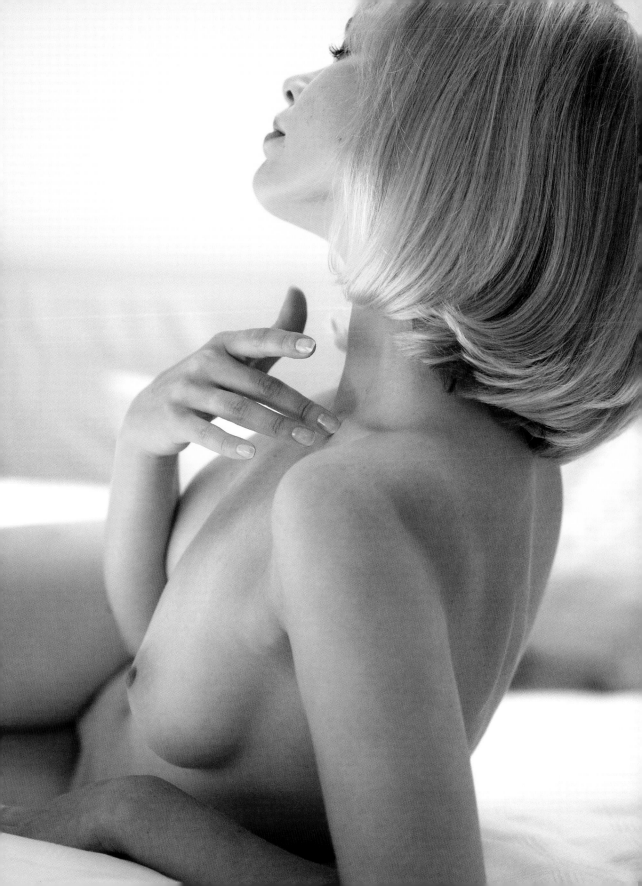

time for yourself

Schedule a regular date with yourself, when you do exactly what you want, and notice how fulfilled you feel afterward. During this time, focus on awakening your senses: spend time with nature, in dance, or in any other activity that makes you feel fully alive. When you look after yourself, you will feel more energized and positive, and more open to trying new things. You will also become a more lively and intuitive partner.

the source of your own ecstasy

Regular time spent alone provides the perfect opportunity to indulge in self-pleasuring. This is the most effective way to discover more about what turns you on or off physically. Tantra encourages and celebrates self-pleasuring as a way to sensitize your own body, making you more open to receiving and giving pleasure. The more you honor your wondrous body, the more someone else will be able to honor it as you would wish.

It is important to regularly nourish and arouse your own body, and not wait for someone else to "do it" for you. Sometimes we are held back by reasons such as a sense of guilt for taking time for your own pleasure, or feelings of shame or embarrassment. Whatever stops you, you need to let go of old patterns of self-denial. You are worth the time and attention from yourself, as well as from a lover. You need to be familiar with your own body, and what makes you feel good, so you can feel comfortable enough to let another pleasure you creatively and intimately. Take time to explore and get to know your own body. The exercises in this book will help you get started.

craving contact

It's perfectly natural to want to be held, caressed, and loved. Everybody needs and craves contact, and many people spend a lot of their lives deprived of nurturing touch. Sometimes men and women go looking for sex just so that they can feel physically connected to another human being.

Keep finding ways to open up and receive more intimate touch. Start by touching yourself, and learning which strokes and pressures are sexiest and most satisfying. Later, this is valuable knowledge to bring to lovemaking. Informed, conscious touch is a master key in opening to the universal energy of love.

10 MINUTE TANTRA

SELF-MASSAGE

Start exploring your physical self by making time to massage your own body with love, as you would wish to be touched by a lover.

1 You can use oil or body lotion. Play some erotic music that makes you feel sexy.
2 Start with just 10 minutes of conscious touch, and find parts of your body that are aching for touch. You could start by simply massaging your arms, face, shoulders, and hands, and move to wherever you want to. Imagine your hands belong to a professional tantric massage therapist who's been sent to you as a gift.
3 Take many deep breaths while you're massaging. This helps to oxygenate the cells of your skin. Let your hands worship your body with passion and creativity.

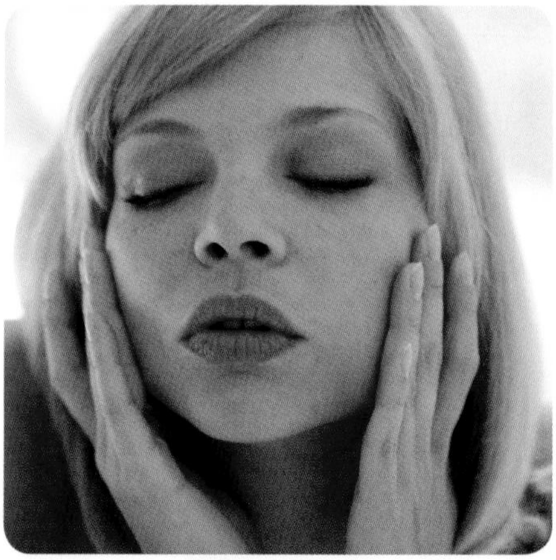

Visual stimulation

Looking at photographs, books, and movies of people pleasuring themselves can be stimulating and educational, so try to find images that appeal to you. Pick up a few different types of erotic art, then watch for some very effective self-pleasuring inspiration.

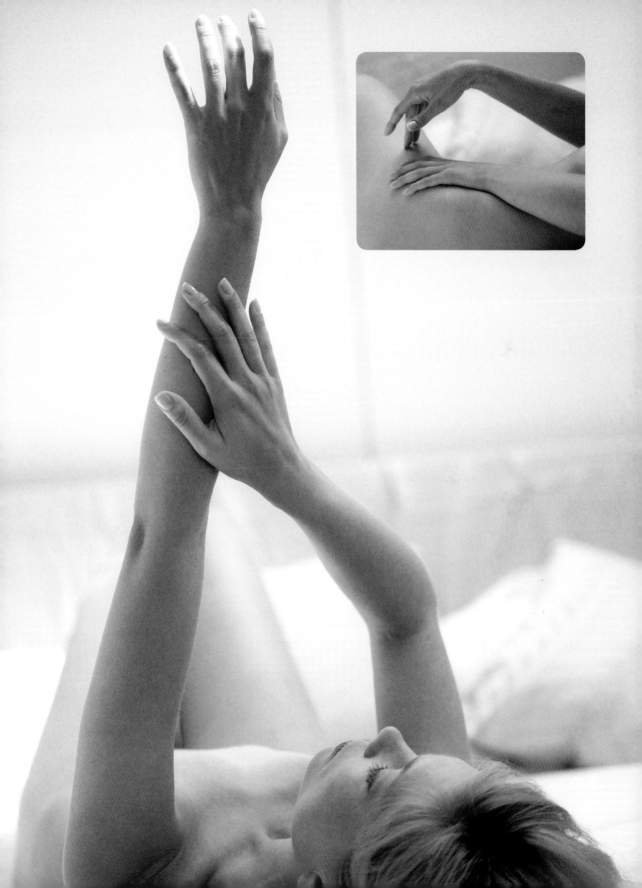

Self-pleasuring for men

In tantric self-pleasuring the goal is to open up the channels for your body energies to start flowing. You become more aware of sensation and how your body responds to pleasure and touch. Your chakras become energized, and you feel fully alive.

activating the root chakra

When a man stimulates his genitals, he is activating his root chakra, creating an inner circular flow of energy. This can take him to a transcendental state of being where he feels fully in the moment, aware of every sensation and feeling. A physical benefit of this energy circulation is that it aids brain function and lymph flow, leading to greater oxygenation of the blood, and more vitality within the whole system. Setting aside regular time for self-pleasuring will cause your root chakra to be open and energized. Get to know your body well, then take this newfound vitality into your relationship with your partner.

enjoying self-pleasuring

It's not unusual for adult men to feel ashamed about masturbation, due to the negative messages they received in childhood. This causes them to inhibit their breathing while they self-pleasure, stifling sounds, and generally contracting the body. The constriction that comes from furtive and secretive masturbation can be carried over into lovemaking with a partner, where some men might never access their full power and ability to give and receive ecstatic pleasure. When you self-pleasure, let yourself go. Make sounds, move your body, and allow yourself to fully enjoy every moment.

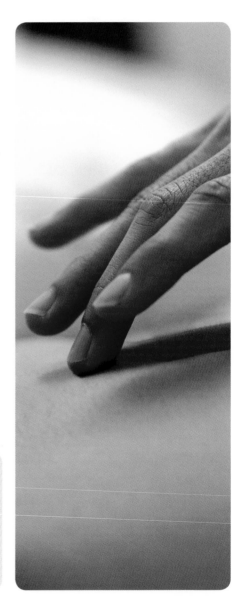

EJACULATION CONTROL

Men generally ejaculate when they masturbate, which not only leaks the seed of life, but also cuts off the energy flow around the sex center. This ends any chance for the expansive pleasure that can be experienced when a man allows sexual energy to spread over his body. There's nothing wrong with ejaculation itself, but to become a truly masterful lover it's useful to learn about ejaculation control (see page 147).

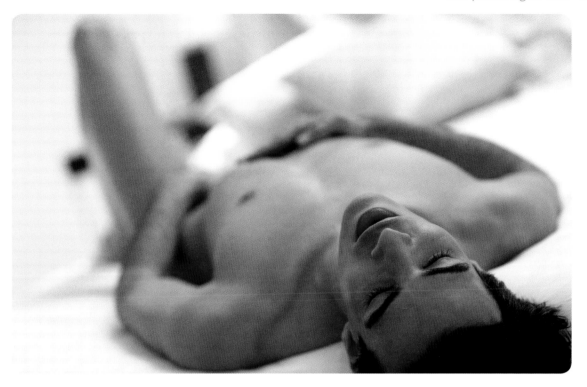

unleash your inner love god

This exercise allows you to reach your full orgasmic potential, and is as much an emotional journey as a physical one. An exercise like this, if done regularly, will become increasingly pleasurable and rewarding. Over time you will discover what touches and techniques are most arousing, allowing yourself to fully open up to orgasmic bliss.

1 Put on some loud, energetic music and get comfortable.

2 Start to rock and gyrate your pelvis, feeling the bones of your hips soften and expand.

3 Touch your lingam and testicles slowly and sensually. Try not to be mechanical or habitual with your touch. Massage your abdomen, and let the heat of sex energy flood your belly.

4 You can allow sounds: moaning, gasping, roaring, anything that expresses your desire for the ultimate orgasm.

5 Undulate your spine, allowing the sex energy to rise up and penetrate your solar plexus. Move spontaneously. It doesn't matter whether you're touching your genitals or not at this point. Move your hands where they want to go.

6 Let your heart be cracked open with the force of sexual heat rising upward. Tune into the connection between sex and heart. What is happening is an orgasm of the heart. Bask in the intensity of this type of pleasure.

7 Be free and expressive. If emotions come, let them— anger, sadness, laughter—don't deny any aspect of your full masculine nature. Shout out, or laugh, as you wish.

8 Imagine that you are penetrating the universe, making love to a giant yoni. Lose yourself completely in lust and desire. Let yourself be swallowed whole by the cosmic yoni.

9 Ejaculation is irrelevant. You have allowed your sexual energy to reach parts of you never reached before. Melt into ecstasy and let waves of bliss flood around your body.

Self-pleasuring for women

The tantric word for vagina is *yoni*, which means "cave of wonder." Wondrous indeed, with its complex layers, the yoni is far more capable of pleasure than most women realize. Self-pleasuring helps you to discover and experience all that your body can give.

pleasuring your yoni

The yoni is a vulnerable area of the body that often does not receive the gentle honor it deserves. This can lead to a desensitisation of the yoni, and sometimes even disenchantment with sex. When it comes to self-pleasuring, women often become preoccupied with their clitoris–unsurprisingly, as it contains approximately 3000 nerve endings, and its sole reason for existing is to feel sexual pleasure. Because of this, some women forget that the whole genital area is capable of deep satisfaction and delight. Through self-pleasuring you can awaken your base chakra, and every nerve-ending in your yoni, and let it flourish and bring joy as it is designed to do.

yoni appreciation

Every woman is unique, her yoni included. If you forge a loving and understanding relationship with your own yoni, your partner will feel more inclined to love and understand it, too. Spend time regularly looking at your yoni with a hand mirror, until you are familiar with its unique character and beauty. Look closely and see the color of your yoni, the contours, and the wetness. Look at your clitoris and your urethral opening, then find your G-spot, beginning just below it. Take deep breaths as you do this, to keep yourself relaxed.

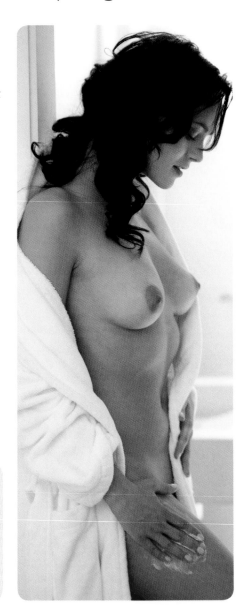

HEALING YOUR YONI

Yoni healings are therapeutic sessions performed by an experienced practitioner, who uses touch, hands-on healing, and talking to guide you to a place of healing. These treatments help women who feel unable to share openly with their lover, are uncomfortable with penetration, are sore from surgery or childbirth, or have felt traumatized by an early, negative sexual experience, teaching them to enjoy their yoni once more.

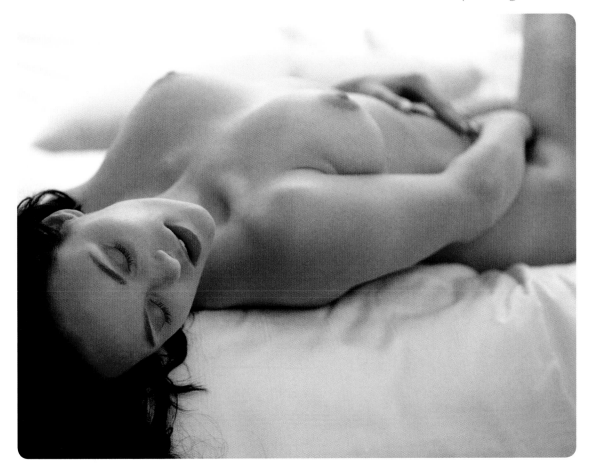

make love to your yoni

Your yoni is designed to bring you immense pleasure in many ways. Take this chance to enjoy your body, and to discover and enjoy areas of your yoni that rarely get any attention, such as your G-spot. Do this meditation regularly, and as you sensitize previously unexplored areas, take this new awareness to your lovemaking.

1 Take a long, sensuous bath or shower. Afterward, massage moisturizing lotions or oils into your body.

2 Put on some erotic music and lay down comfortably.

3 Begin by touching and caressing the outside of your yoni with your fingers. Touch yourself as if you've never felt the gateway to your cave of wonder before.

4 Massage your labia slowly and sensually, noticing and relaxing into the different sensations that arise.

5 Take time to caress and titillate your yoni, and move to gently stimulate your clitoris. Take your time and tune in to how your body reacts as you pleasure your yoni.

6 Feel just below your urethral opening (located just above your vaginal opening). This is the start of your prostate, or G-spot. Gently rub this spongy area, and begin to sensitize it. You may feel a need to urinate: this is normal, and will pass.

7 Orgasm if you wish, or simply enjoy the feelings of blissful pleasure that wash over your body.

Wake up your sexuality

Tantricas regard sexual union as a doorway to higher consciousness, and we find the key to that door through awakening and stimulating the senses. Dancing is one of the best ways to do this, as it ignites a powerful sensual force, called "kundalini energy."

stimulating your sex drive

Tantra encourages you to wake up every aspect of your sexuality, so you can experience all the joys of a rich and fulfilling life. Self-pleasure is one way to awaken your sexual energy, as is spending time in meditation with your partner. You can also wake up your sexuality through any type of sensual physical activity. Dancing is an energizing way to remind yourself of what it feels like when love and self-respect are fully present. Through simple erotic steps, you fire up your sex drive, and stimulate your sense of sound, touch, and sight.

EXPERIENCE KUNDALINI ENERGY

Kundalini is a life force energy that is sourced from the *kunda*, a gland in the sacrum. It lies dormant at the base of your spine just behind your sacrum. Everyone has the capacity to awaken his or her kundalini energy. When this happens, it begins to rise through the body, curling like a snake, stimulating the chakras until it penetrates the crown of your head and bursts forth, lighting up the cosmos.

dancing for an invisible lover

Try this meditation alone to awaken your sexuality and desire. As you dance and allow your body to move as it wants to, notice how your energy levels rise and you become more alert. Caress your body and become aware of the softness of your skin, and how touch makes you feel. Your body is designed to be sexy, so let it be sexy!

1 Put on some erotic dance music (see Resources page 184). Start to move as if dancing for a lover who is watching you.

2 Picture in your mind whoever it is you desire to represent your "lover." It can be an actual partner or an imagined one.

3 Begin to remove your clothing slowly and sensually. Gradually reveal more and more of yourself to your adoring lover. He or she is infatuated with every inch of your body.

4 When you are naked, dance with full movement, revelling in your own beauty. Free your hips, letting the kundalini snake awaken from its slumber. Allow the potent sexual energy to rise like the flames of a fire. Undulate your spine,

feeling the kundalini energy firing up every vertebra on its way up your central channel.

5 After the dancing, lie down, and imagine your lover blowing a warm breath gently over your body.

6 Caress your body, imagining the hands of your lover stroking you with desire. Let the passion increase, holding nothing back. Touch your face, hair, and parts of your body that never get touched. Caress your genitals with love.

7 Allow the hands of your imaginary lover to transport you to a place of orgasmic bliss. After the climactic waves have died down, rest in peaceful serenity.

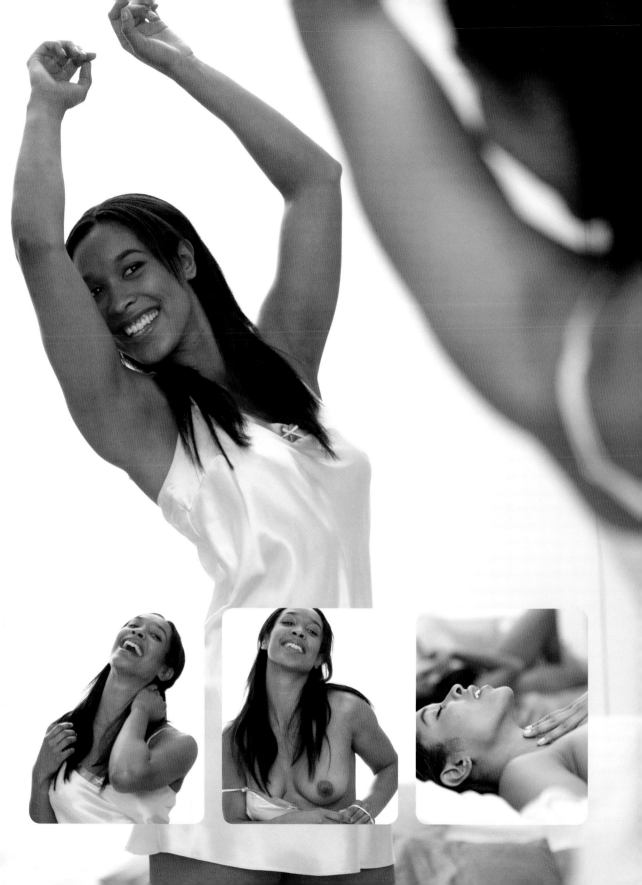

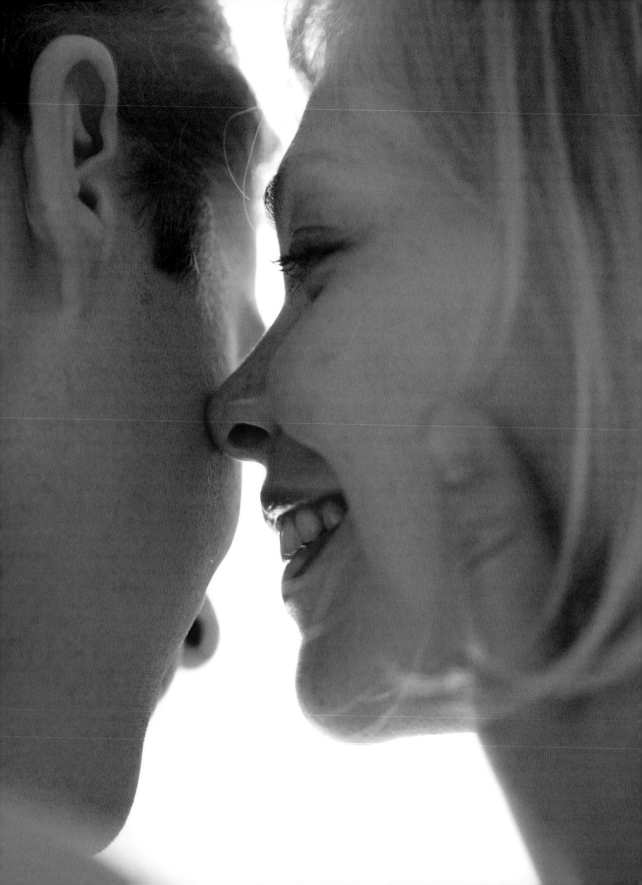

5

ENGAGING THROUGH CELEBRATION

Make it a priority to celebrate life with your partner on a regular basis. Connecting through time spent in nature, dance, and imaginative play will clear your mind and heart, add intimacy to your relationship, and reinvigorate your sex life. Your relationship and your sex life will thrive from this new sensual joyfulness.

Connecting with nature

Nature has much to teach us in the ways of the human body and the subtle energy realms that operate deep within it. The meditations that follow provide a gateway into the divine world of nature, a world of sensuous beauty that you can enjoy and celebrate with your partner.

becoming aware of natural energy

People are intrinsically connected with nature. Like leaves and birds and stones, all humans are made up of energy molecules vibrating at different speeds. We all generate cosmic energy. It is important that you spend time connecting with nature, on your own and with your partner. As you become aware of the vibrational energy that surrounds you, and how you feel when you are close to natural energy, you can bring this heightened sensory awareness to your sexual relationship.

bringing nature into your relationship

In our modern world we spend a lot of time inside our homes and offices, and most of us spend too little time in the great outdoors. We forget that underneath our clothes, we are instinctual creatures, naked and primitive in our essential nature.

Spending time with your loved one outside reconnects you with your primal temperament. Space, fresh air, water, and weather bring you closer to your true self and your partner. You come alive when you connect with nature. It is extremely peaceful to walk in nature, and there is more space in which to share and express issues that may be difficult to communicate at other times. During a relaxed stroll, concerns or problems can be aired more easily. It's almost as if the wind, sunlight, trees, and ocean hear our thoughts, too, and carry them away.

EROTIC SHAPES IN NATURE

Sensual shapes and erotic forms are to be found everywhere in nature. You can see trees like bodies and flowers like yonis. This is because nature and sex are closely linked. Bring sensual nature into your home to convey its peaceful and seductive atmosphere.

a natural relationship

This is a practical way to teach your soul how to connect deeply with nature. If you allow the energy and power of nature into your heart, you will be friends for life.

1 Go into a garden or park. Walk around and wait for a leaf to "call" you to it.

2 Take this leaf into your hand and feel its temperature and weight. Look at the leaf's color and texture. Gaze deep into the intricate patterns of its veins and feel its life-force energy vibrating in your hand. See if the leaf has any message for you.

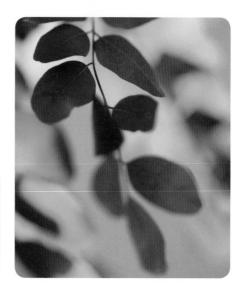

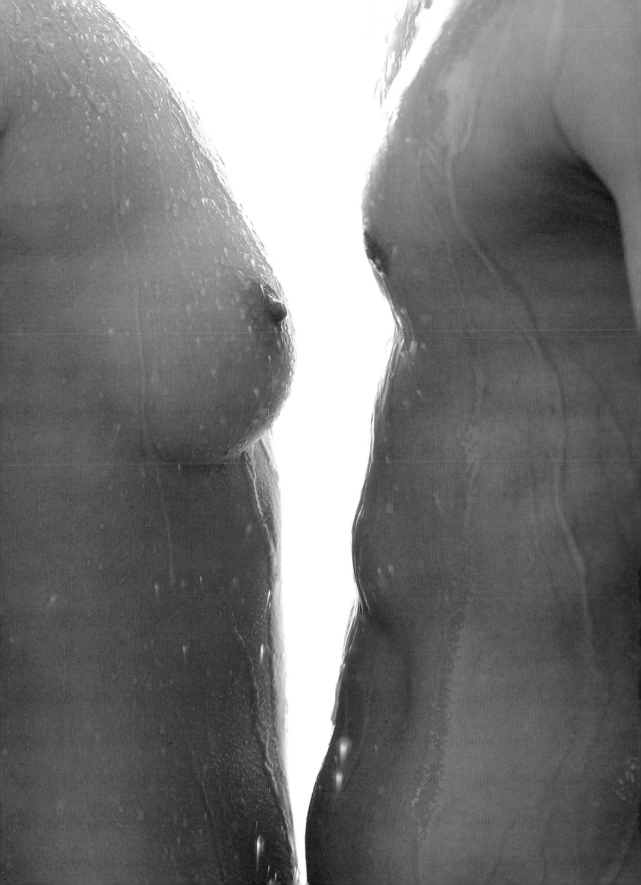

blindfold in nature

For this meditation you need to be in a quiet, private garden or area of countryside where you won't be disturbed. Choose a sunny day, if possible. This meditation calls for trust; the blindfolded partner trusts the other to keep them safe. This slow, gentle meditation subtly heightens the senses.

1 Perform the opening ceremony (see page 12).

2 Blindfold your partner, then lead him or her out to the garden or quiet area, slowly and sensitively. Take care of your partner so that they can let go into the meditation and experience the ecstasy of meeting nature in an intimate way.

3 Guide them slowly to a flower, tree, or fruit. Take their hands and place them on it. Let your partner feel, smell, or taste the discovery, if they would like.

4 Remove the blindfold and let your partner see what they've been feeling. Allow each other the time to look. Soften your gaze and look with yin vision (see page 110).

5 Blindfold your partner again to repeat the meditation one or more times and then swap turns. You can take as long as you like to savor each new sensual discovery.

6 Return inside or to the area where you started, and perform the closing ceremony (see page 12).

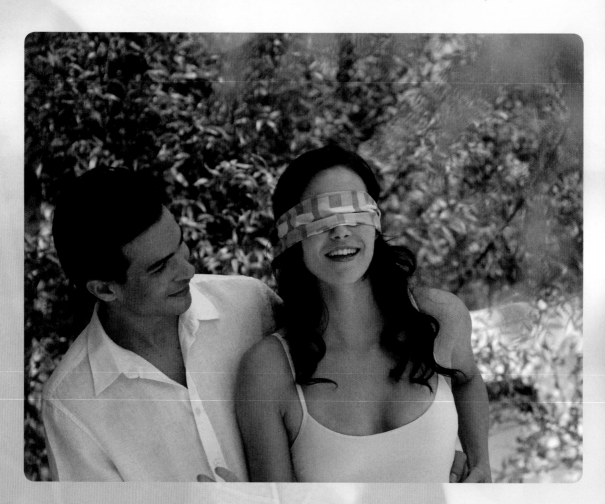

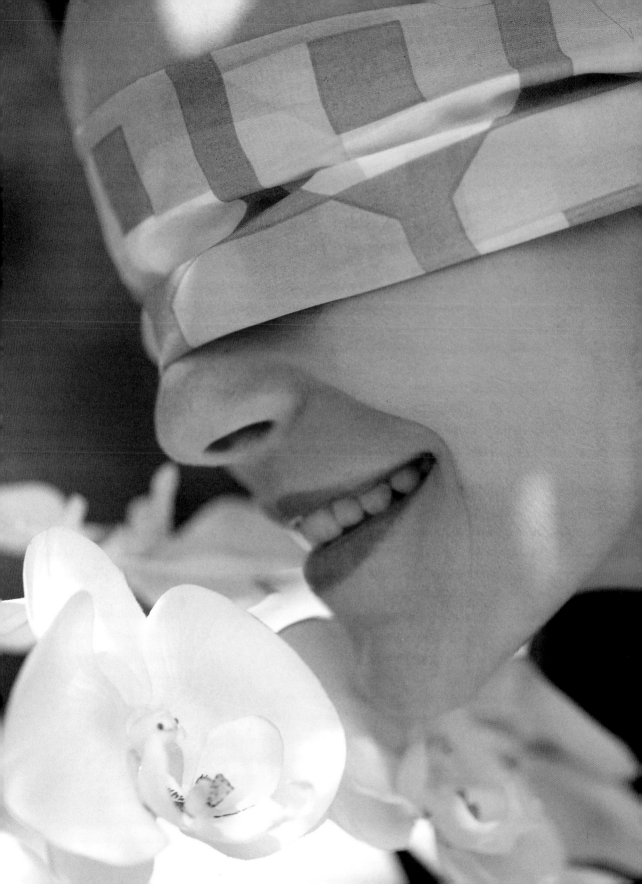

Dancing together

Everybody can dance. Regardless of age or background, we can all learn how to let music move our bodies. Dancing awakens the chakras, energizes you, and makes you feel alive. Sensual dancing such as stripping taps into this heightened awareness, enriching sexuality.

communication through dance

Dancing creates sensual intimacy, and acts as a potent remedy for unresolved issues within the relationship. When dancing, lovers can communicate feelings they have about each other in a non-verbal way. It is intrinsically sensual, and activates positive mood-enhancing brain chemicals that flood the whole body via the cardiovascular system. When the body is moving spontaneously, the mind lessens its hold, allowing for a channel of communication that exists beyond words.

free up your pelvis

Dancing is another way to activate your kundalini energy (see page 66), a powerful sexual energy originating at the back of the sacrum. When moving to music, it can shimmer its way up your spine, energizing your chakras and opening the crown chakra, leading to a heightened state of awareness.

If your hips are rigid and the sacrum held tight, your kundalini energy will lay dormant. Dancing increases your ability to move your hips separately from the rest of your body, encouraging them to express their own personality, and prompting your kundalini energy to uncurl and start to rise.

An additional benefit of loosening your pelvis is that both of you will increase your physical flexibility in lovemaking. A man will also find he is more able to gain control over ejaculation.

There are many dance classes that you can join to learn how to get your pelvis moving, from salsa to ballroom dancing, but if you are a little self-conscious to start, you can let your hips come out of the closet in private at home. Simply play some great music at a loud volume and get moving.

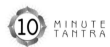

10 MINUTE TANTRA

WARM-UP DANCE

At the end of a busy day, and perhaps before a longer meditation, spend a few minutes doing this energizing warm-up dance.

1 Put on music that inspires you to dance. Let your body and limbs move spontaneously, freeing up your energy.
2 Shake out any stress held in your body. Make sounds to release tension—feel free to let go, and to shout, laugh, or sing.
3 Dance until your edges disappear and you've gone beyond rational thought.
4 At the end of the warm up, stand still, and feel the energy throughout your body.

RITUAL DANCES

Indigenous cultures throughout India, Asia, Africa, the Americas, and the Middle East, among others, have used dance as a form of worship for millennia. Letting your body be moved by universal energy can instigate an experience of *satori*—a Buddhist term meaning "sudden enlightenment" or "transcendental awakening." Through ecstatic dance one enters an altered state of consciousness. This form of movement is sometimes called "trance dance."

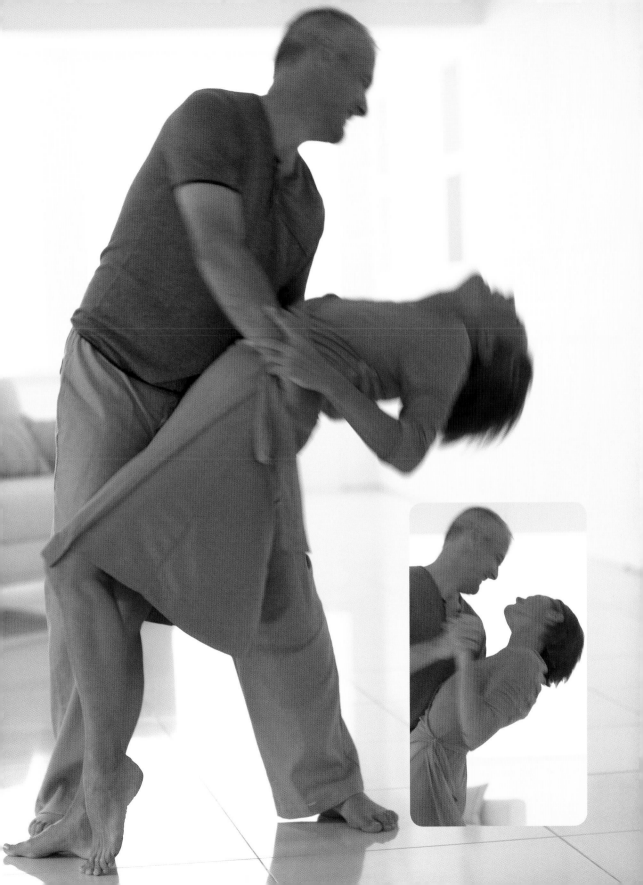

kundalini rising

This is a wonderful way to encourage your kundalini energy to wake up. Dance this meditation together, and see how it encourages you to connect. Notice how your bodies begin to move together, as your kundalini snakes awaken and move upward through your bodies. Have fun, and allow yourselves to laugh and let go.

1 Choose some music that you and your partner both enjoy dancing to. Sexy salsa music will inspire your hips to move!

2 Dance back-to-back, connecting at your sacrums.

3 Picture the kundalini snake waking up and unraveling upward from the base of your spine. Move in a serpent-like fashion, letting your spine be fluid and free. Make sure you don't lean back on your partner—stay upright.

4 Raise your arms—let them be a conduit for universal energy. Feel cosmic energy pour down through your body merging with the fire rising from your base chakra. The two energy flows are spiralling up and down, swirling around each other like a double helix. Revel in a sense of pure vibration.

5 At the end of the music, turn and face each other, placing your foreheads together, connecting at the sixth chakra (see page 20). Breathe, and feel your energies merging together.

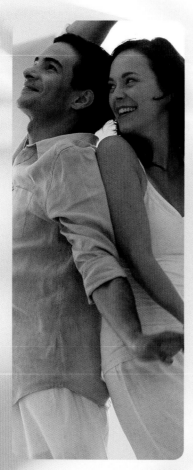
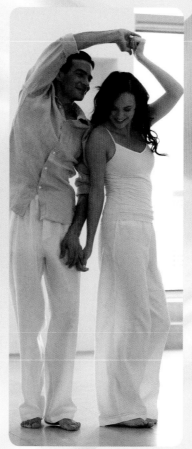
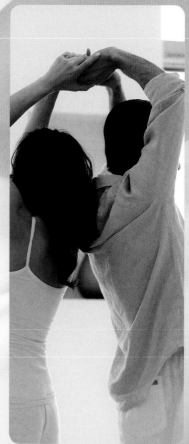

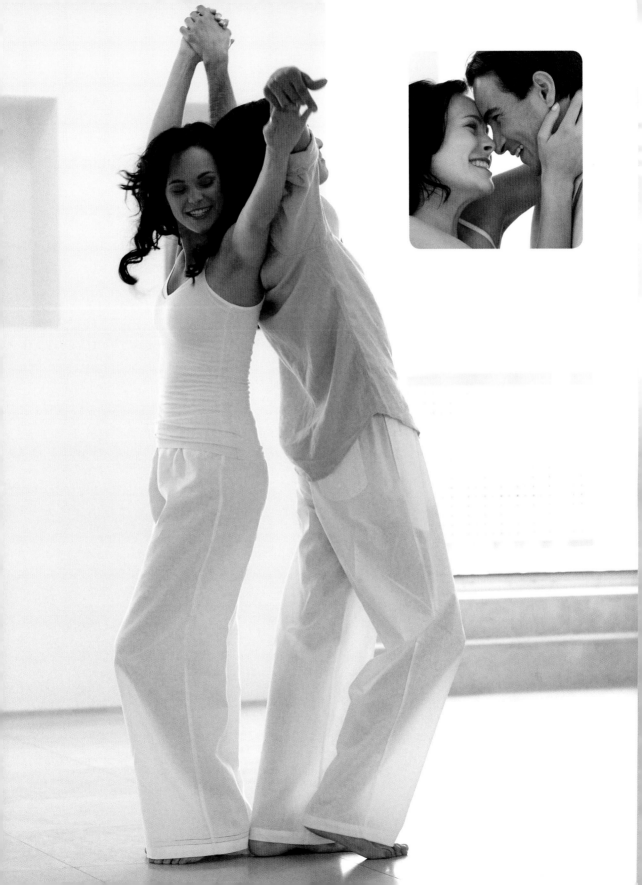

sexy stripping

The more you dance for each other, the more comfortable you and your lover will become in delighting one another with any newly-acquired seduction techniques, both on the dance floor and in bed. Choose a piece of sexy dance music lasting about twenty minutes and begin exploring the exciting realm of strip dancing, as you "perform" together.

1 Namaste your partner (see page 10).

2 Dance opposite each other, seducing each other with your eyes. As the energy builds, the woman removes an item of her partner's clothing. Then the man removes a piece of the woman's clothing. Take your time and don't rush.

3 Take turns removing one another's clothes, until you're dancing completely naked. (Try not to leave the man dancing in his socks—or if you do, laugh with him, not at him!)

4 Enjoy each other's natural beauty. Notice if you are feeling self-conscious; if so, breathe, and let your feelings become part of the energy and passion of the dance.

5. Allow yourselves to laugh and be natural—this should be fun! The more relaxed you become, the more comfortable you will be with trying new techniques and finding what works best.

6 After the dance, come together in a warm embrace, feeling a deep sense of gratitude for your playful partner.

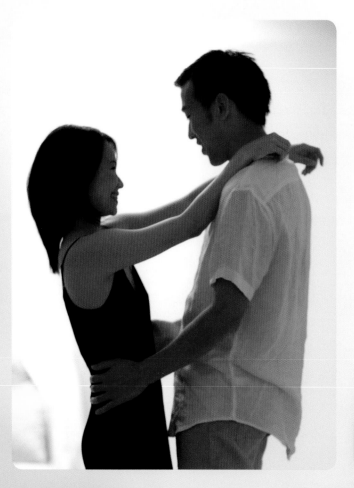

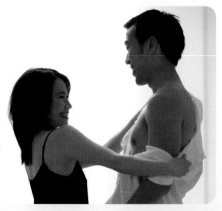

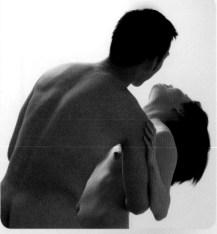

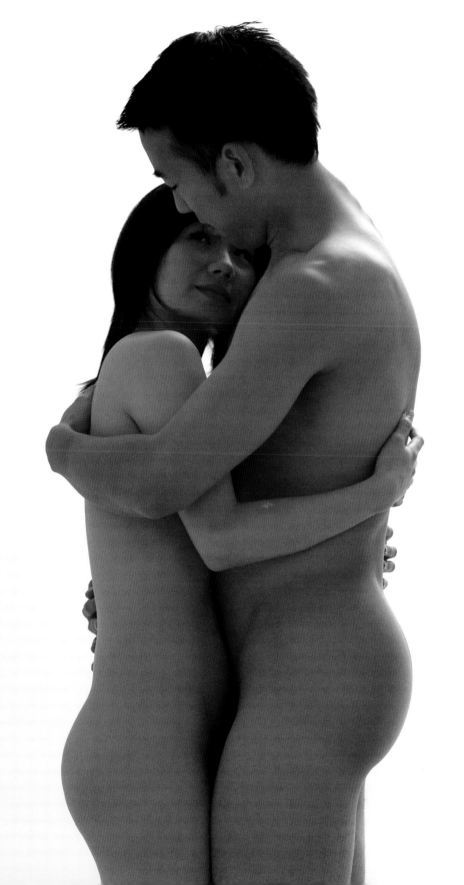

Laughter and play

Playing with your partner in a light-hearted way can re-ignite the flame of desire. Tantra is profound and transforming, but it's not a serious business. These games are for you and your partner to enjoy, and to help you access the sexy power that is generated through play.

unleash your imagination

The imagination is an aspect of your unconscious mind, and it plays a fundamental role in relationships. A large part of sexual attraction arises through a kind of creative process within the lover, meaning that what goes on in your mind is often more important than what is actually true of your beloved. Because of this, we can project any fantasy onto our interactions with our partner. This facility, unique to humans, can be used to great advantage in erotic play and sex games.

Think of your imagination as a muscle that you can either use regularly, or let it atrophy through neglect. We "imagine" our life into actuality. "As we think, so we are," the saying goes. We could take this further and theorize; "As we play, so we are." The beauty of imagination is that it belongs to you. It's your own private world that you can manifest into reality, if you choose.

the game of life

Sharing that private world with a loving partner is a privilege, and helps to generate feelings of profound intimacy within the relationship. Playing, imagining, and laughing together with your partner is a wonderful way to loosen up, and lighten up. You may think you are not in the mood for sex, especially after a busy, tiring day, but you still want to spend time with your partner; play can give you this, and who knows where it can lead. Imaginative play can help you leave adult responsibilities behind, and leave the path clear for intimacy.

Laughing also stimulates circulation in your body–not to mention attraction, arousal, and playful eroticism. Think of life as a game sometimes, and you'll find your relationship becomes more sensual, intimate, and enjoyable.

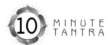

10 MINUTE TANTRA

ENERGIZING LAUGHTER

Laughter is addictive–the more you do it, the more you want to do it. Laughing regularly is a good way to engage with your "inner child" and stay connected with your partner. Focus on letting your bodies relax as you start, so that you can be fully abandoned.

1 Lie next to each other. Stretch and yawn for five minutes.
2 Laugh from the belly for five minutes. If you have difficulty beginning, just start by saying the words, "Ha, ha, ha."
3 As your body quakes with laughter you will feel your pelvis softening and opening, and your genitals responding to the vibration. It feels very sexy to laugh if you notice what's happening in your base chakra.
4 Lie quietly together after the laughter has died down, and experience the subtle, shimmering sensation that you feel in your body as a stream of sexual energy that energizes your whole being.

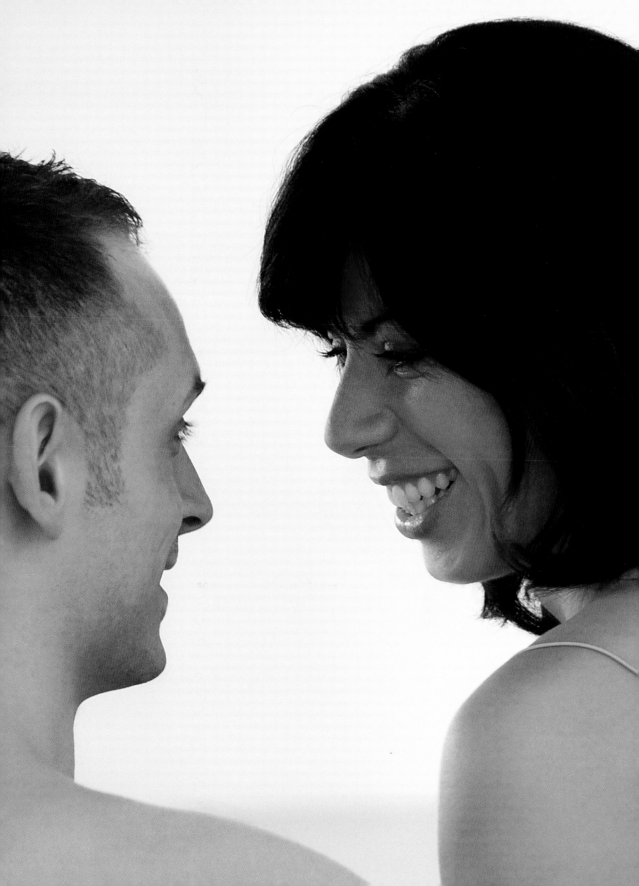

embracing the other

Most people love to play dress-up and this exercise takes the game to a whole new level. Gender swapping can be liberating and for some, a surprising turn-on. This meditation will no doubt give you a few insights into what makes your partner tick. Celebrate each other's creativity and spontaneity and allow yourselves to have fun and laugh.

1   The man dresses as a woman, and the woman dresses as a man. The man can wear makeup. Think about what defines the other person and use props to help you to feel as if you've stepped into the role totally. Have fun. Pretend you're getting into costume for a play and enjoy the process.

2   Put on some funky music and dance with each other, fully embodying the male and the female within your dancing.

3   The man sits down and the woman dances for her lover, impersonating him in her movements. Incorporate his mannerisms into your dance. Think the thoughts that he would think, feel the music like he would.

4   Swap, so that the man dances for his lover, embodying her characteristics and demonstrating them in the dance. Have fun with it—exaggerate the idiosyncracies of your partner and if your audience of one laughs, enjoy it.

5   Put on some sexy dance music. The woman sits down. The man seduces his partner with his dance and then begins to make love to her still in role. He is playing the seductress.

6   As you both slowly discard your clothing, retain the feeling of what it's like to make love as the opposite gender.

7   When you've finished making love, namaste your partner still naked (see page 10). Feel gratitude for your partner's willingness to explore his or her sexuality with you, to play and let go.

CROSS-DRESSING PLAY

It's common for men to feel some resistance toward cross-dressing. This isn't surprising when you realize how manipulated we are by the male and female stereotypes thrown at us from childhood and from the media. Perhaps men are afraid that it might trigger some latent homosexual tendency.

Tantra teaches that a man's fear of exploring his feminine side is wholly unnecessary. The truth is, the more a man can come to accept and enjoy his feminine side the more he'll be able to step into his full masculine power, celebrating his magnificent yang male energy. Men with this type of strength and self-confidence make the best, most confident, and intuitive lovers.

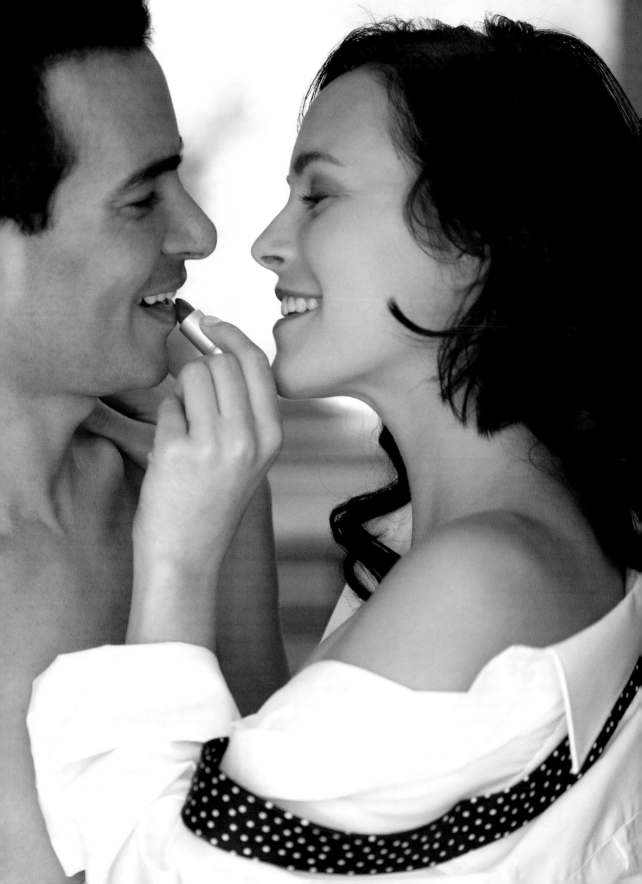

lion's play

In tantra we honor both our animal as well as our spiritual natures. It's actually not possible to have one without the other—we wouldn't be human. The following exercise gives you a chance to let your inner animal out to play. It's a fun way to loosen up. Don't think about it too much; jump in, and have fun.

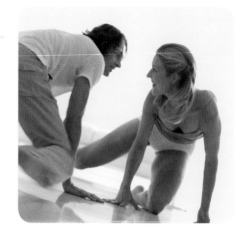

1 Namaste each other (see page 10).

2 Become lions and begin to crawl around the room. Think about the characteristics of lions and start to embody the spirit of the animals.

3 Make lion sounds such as growling and purring. Sniff different things in the room as if you are discovering them for the first time. Allow yourself to become fully animal. Do this for five minutes or so.

4 Come face to face, as two lions meeting. Imagine that you feel instantly threatened. Let territorial feelings arise, such as wariness and mistrust. Prowl around each other, growling with suspicion.

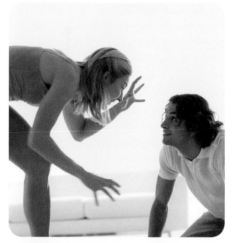

5 One of you becomes slightly more aggressive. Come up onto your knees and push on each other's hands with equal pressure, roaring loudly. Let your anger be expressed in the roar. Find strength in your body and become wild and feral. Do this for at least five minutes.

6 At some point, let the fight die down naturally, as you realize that you both possess equal strength and don't want to fight anymore.

7 Start to smell and lick each other, curious to find out more about this fellow creature. Crawl around your partner, getting to know each other.

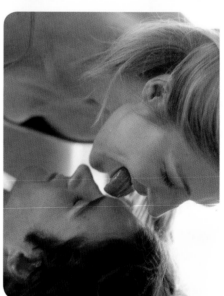

8 Curl up on the floor together as two big cats, exhausted and spent of all energy, but happy that you've made a new and powerful friend.

9 After resting for a while, slowly stand up and come back into your human form. Let your breathing become relaxed and calm.

10 Namaste each other to complete the meditation.

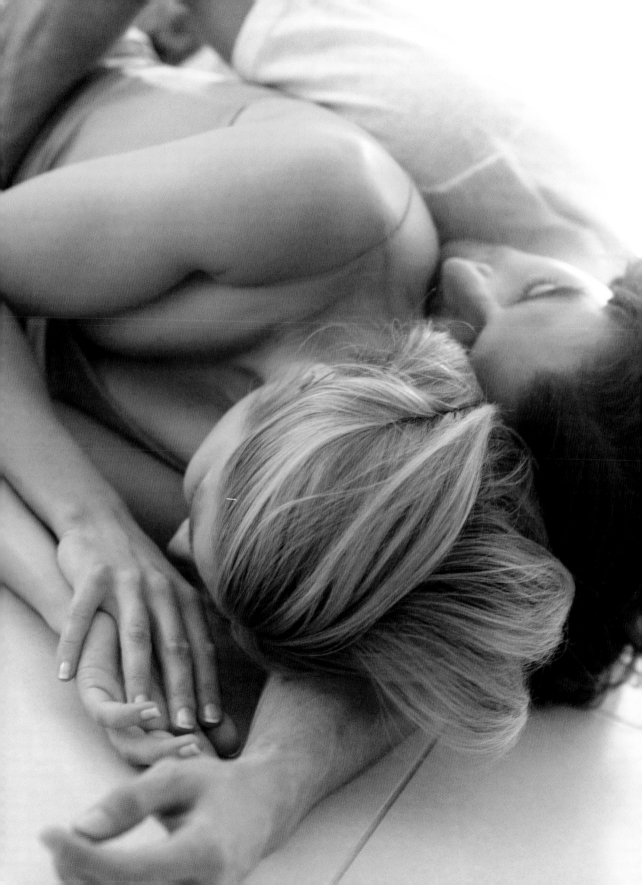

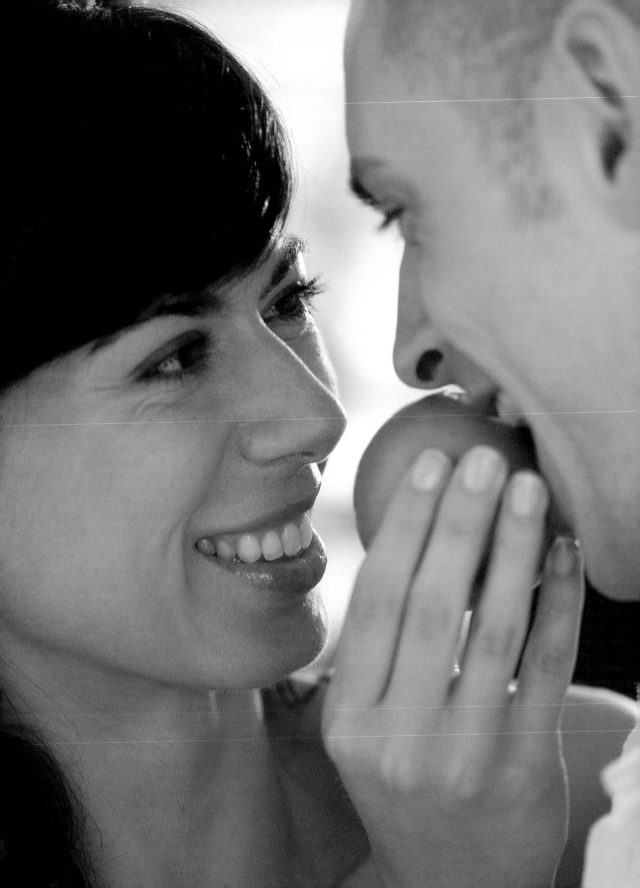

6

ENGAGING THROUGH THE SENSES

As we work with our senses through tantra, they become increasingly heightened. Plan specific times to explore the subtle dimensions of smell, taste, sight, sound, and touch with your partner—you'll be entering a sensual world that will draw you deeper into its mystery on every part of the journey.

Scent

All your senses can act as portals into an expanded state of consciousness, but the most evocative of all is your sense of smell. A scent can transport your mind to a different place and mindset, and can relax or energize you, ready for tantric play.

the power of scent

The human nose is a highly sensitive organ that can detect the difference between more than 10,000 chemicals. Our sense of smell is so closely linked to the brain that it has the potential to send us into altered states of consciousness.

Smells travel on tiny olfactory nerves straight to the "hypothalamus," a gland in the brain responsible for regulating dozens of bodily functions, among which are hunger, thirst, sleeping and waking, sexual arousal, and emotions such as anger and happiness. The message carried in an odor also travels to the "hippocampus," the part of the brain responsible for memory, which explains why smells recall the past so vividly.

pheromones and arousal

According to ancient tantric teachings, smell is the sense that ignites sexual energy. Chemistry between lovers is a complex thing; just as you can be attracted or repelled by the way another person looks, you can also be turned on or off by their smell.

When you are aroused you emit "pheromones," chemicals that elicit a natural behavioral response in another member of the same species. There are many different types of these subtle, yet powerful scent chemicals. If you are interested sexually in a particular partner, you start to emit certain pheromones. These pheromones can be appealing to the man or woman you want to seduce, or they can have the opposite effect.

Pay attention to the subtle messages you are receiving through your sense of smell when you find yourself up close and personal with a potential lover. The effect of your partner's scent can be a crucial factor in the success of a sexual relationship.

☯ Enhance your personal scent

The scent you emanate can be affected positively or negatively by your diet, so it's important to give thought to what you eat and drink. Eat wholesome, organic food and avoid garlic. Drink plenty of water and refrain from indulging in large amounts of alcohol. Use organic body products scented with natural plant aromas, rather than synthetic fragrances.

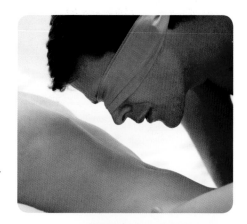

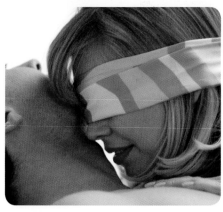

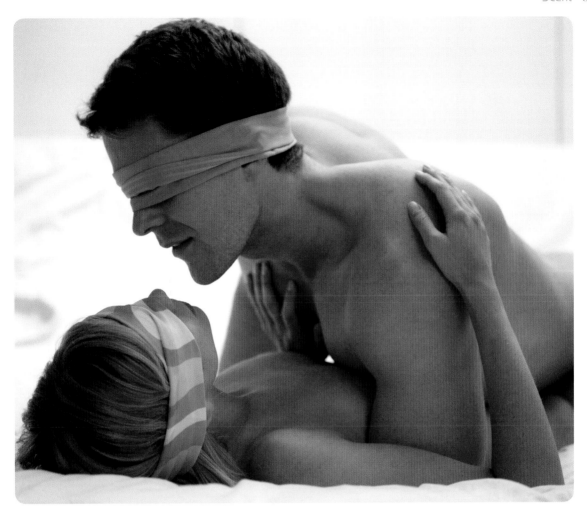

the scent of love

This is a wonderful way to pay awareness to each other's scents. Stay alert to the mysterious and subtle nuances of scent, as your bodies discover each other through this powerful way. Notice how you react. Your body will become aware of your partner in a new way, as you both emit sexy pheromones.

1 Take a long, luxurious shower together. Use non-synthetic products that won't mask your natural scent.

2 Put on some dance music. One of you lie down while the other dances naked in front of you. Then change places.

3 Both lie down, and one of you put on a blindfold.

4 If you are the blindfolded partner, investigate the body of your beloved, using only your nose. Include all areas of the body. Indulge in this olfactory feast for at least five minutes.

5 Swap around so the other partner is blindfolded and takes a turn to discover their lover. Take your time, and smell parts of your partner's body you've never dared to smell before. Relax and enjoy this sensory exploration.

6 Both put on blindfolds and enter into lovemaking.

arousing your sense of smell

This is an easy tantric meditation that is a good starting point if you are new to tantra. Notice how the ritual brings new energy to the process of smelling and tasting, and how your senses become enhanced in the process. When you move in to lovemaking, continue to experience the closeness you created, and enjoy your heightened senses.

1 Perform the opening ceremony (see page 12).

2 The woman gently blindfolds her partner and asks him to sit or lie down in a relaxed and comfortable position.

3 Take three tissues and pour a few drops of different essential oil on to each tissue. Aim for a variety of scents.

4 Slowly waft the first tissue close to the nose of your partner, allowing him to smell deeply the scent of the oil. Repeat with the next two scents, pausing between each.

5 Next, take a piece of fruit, and squeeze it gently so that it emits its aroma. Let your partner smell the fruit. Sensitively place the fruit on his lips, which he parts, allowing you to gently move the fruit into his mouth. He slowly takes in the taste a and texture, relishing the subtle nuances of the flavour.

6 He then lets the two senses of smell and taste combine for an ecstatic olfactory explosion. He will notice that his senses are heightened and the flavour of the fruit intensified.

7 Change around, so the woman experiences the smells and tastes. Choose a different fruit to experiment with.

8 Remove the blindfold and make love if you desire, smelling and tasting each other to your hearts content. Become lost in the exquisite rhapsody of smells and tastes merging.

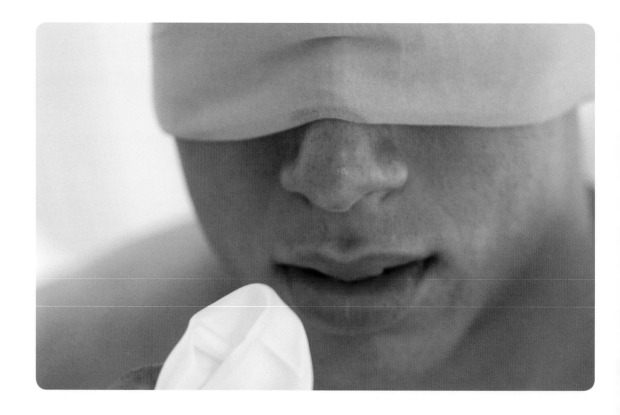

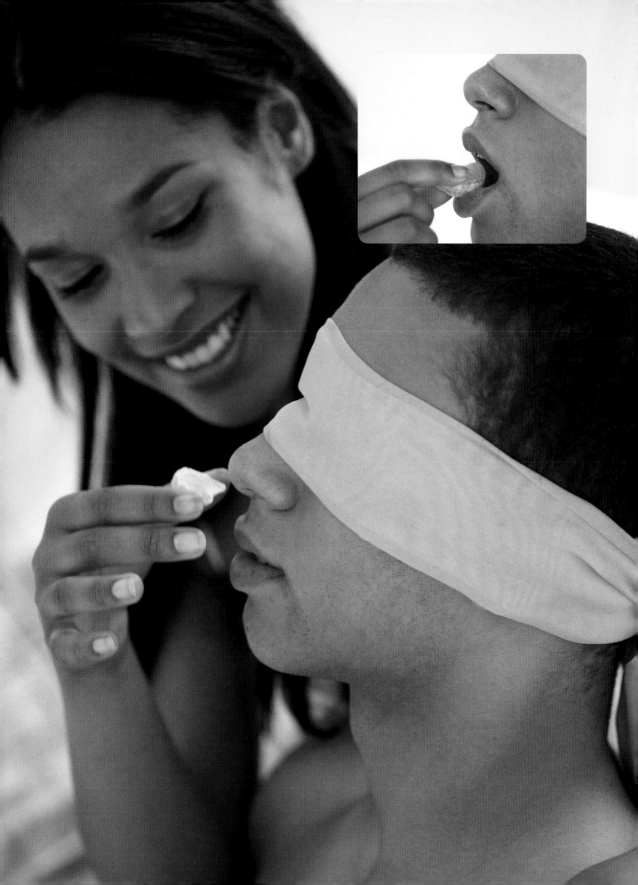

Taste

Food and drink can provide some of the greatest sensory pleasures, but few of us take time to enjoy what we eat. In tantra, we encourage you to savor each bite, and to think about incorporating taste into different areas of your life, including meditation with your partner.

the language of taste

Human beings are limited to six descriptions of taste: sweet, sour, salty, bitter, astringent, and pungent. But if we examine each of these tastes separately, letting the delicate qualities of each imbibe us with their essence, the nuances become more noticeable. The human tongue has about 10,000 taste buds that are there to keep us interested in eating. As you taste a food, think about its flavor, and why it is appealing or not. Find the foods that both your tastebuds and your body respond to, and learn to savor them as a sensory treat that you deserve regularly. View each meal as a time for healthful indulgence.

taste and the body

New cells in your body are constructed from the nutrients you take in daily: you literally are what you eat. In turn, the various smells and tastes of our bodies reflect what we consume. Semen, for example, can taste very different depending on what a man has been eating and drinking. The same is true for saliva and, of course, the secretions from a woman's yoni.

Your body reflects your inner levels of health and wellbeing. In tantric lovemaking not only do we become acutely aware of how our partner feels, we increase our sensitivity to them in other ways, such as how they taste. Developing a high degree of consciousness in this area can deepen your connection.

As you refine your sense of taste through tantric practice, the awareness about what you eat happens naturally, with no feelings of guilt attached. You simply feel the joy of tasting pure and untainted food, and become more discerning in your choices. Fresh, healthy food makes you feel good in many ways, and awakens your sensitivity to all kinds of pleasure.

☙ Eating blindfold

In tantra we refine the senses through bringing our undivided attention to every activity we engage in. One of the most effective ways of honing and refining one particular sense is to deactivate others so that we can more fully explore the sense we're aiming to become more intimate with.

Eating while blindfolded allows you to concentrate fully on flavors and texture without being distracted by sight, sound, or touch. The sense of smell is important in augmenting taste, and you will want to fully utilize it, so get your nose involved.

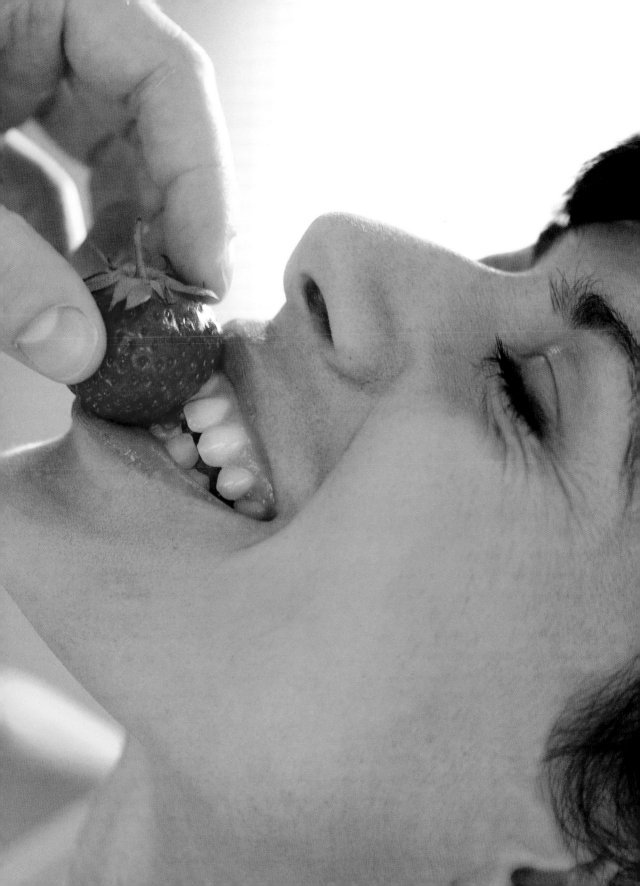

arousing your sense of taste

Take time to taste and savor delicious foods together. When you are blindfolded and deprived of the sense of sight, your sense of taste will flourish. Prepare a plate of bite-sized morsels of wholesome foods, like banana, almonds, berries, melon, apple, coconut, raisins, avocado, or plum. Include a glass of high-quality organic wine.

1 Perform the opening ceremony (see page 12).

2 The woman reclines on comfortable cushions and puts on a blindfold. The man prepares the plate of food and wine.

3 The man feeds his partner with one piece of fruit in turn, letting her luxuriate in the taste and texture. Allow her to really take her time to explore the sensations arising from the discovery of these delectable morsels.

4 The man gently pours a little wine into his partner's mouth. Let the fragrance and flavor of the wine fill your whole body and let yourself "become" the wine. Feel a sense of reverential respect as you drink the wine.

5 Change around, so the man is now blindfolded. The woman introduces her partner to the food and wine, and he takes his turn to "discover" each bite as if he has never tasted food and wine before.

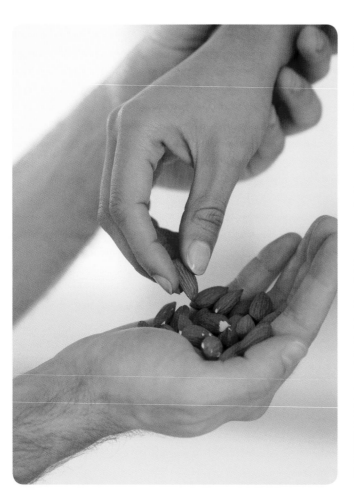

A PASSION FOR WINE

A fine organic wine has often been grown, fermented, and bottled with loving care. Many wine makers consider their beloved creations to be works of art. See if you can taste the passion in every sip you take. You may even be able to sense the spirit of the vintner in the wine.

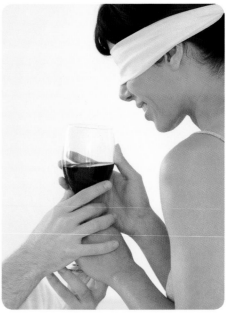

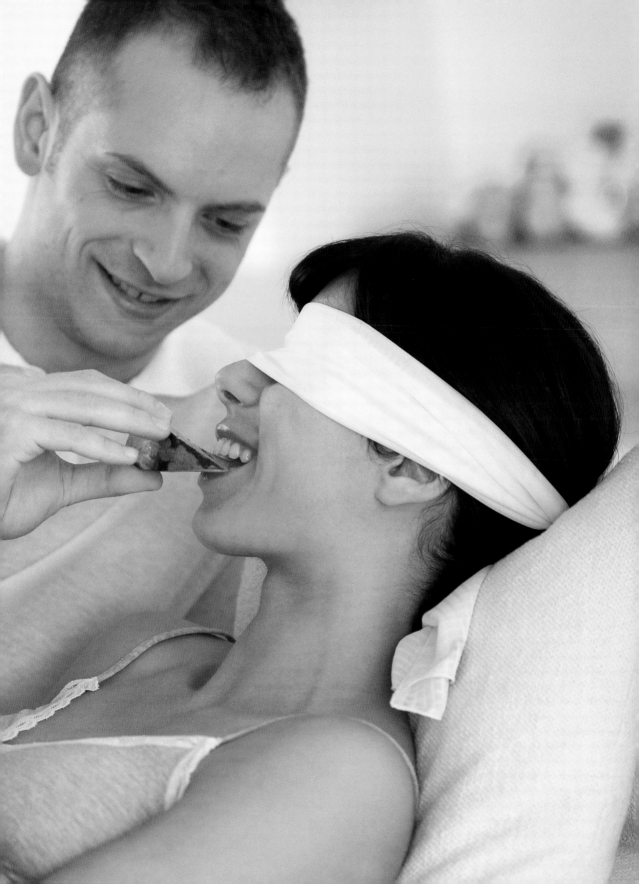

a sensual feast

This meditation uses taste and smell as a doorway to ecstasy. It is ideal as foreplay or after-play. Practicing this meditation naked will enhance the experience, and you can blindfold your partner to add still further intimacy. Eat from each other's bodies—use your lingam as a spoon, and serve dessert from your breasts.

1 Prepare a comfortable temple space, with large cushions to recline on. Light candles and ensure the room is warm. Prepare a tray of morsels of delicious, good quality food.

2 Shower together using only natural products.

3 Feed your partner slowly and sensuously, allowing time for them to smell and taste each bite. Be playful—you can use various parts of your body for feeding.

4 Change over regularly. Every so often you may wish to whisper the Shiva Sutra to your partner: "When eating or drinking, become the taste of food or drink, and be filled."

5 This meal should be unhurried and relaxed, with both of you taking turns and being experimental with how you serve the food. You won't eat as much as you normally do, and the sensual playfulness of this meditation can slip into lovemaking whenever you desire.

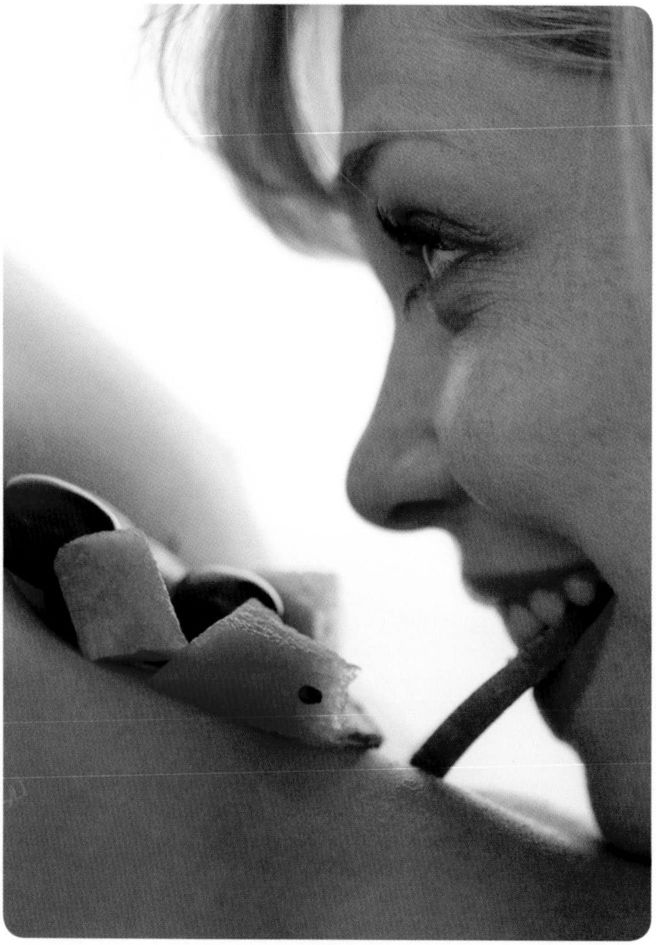

Choosing foods for your meal

Prepare an exotic meal that includes a variety of flavors and scents, including salty, sweet, and spicy choices. Avoid foods with garlic as it has an anaesthetic quality that can inhibit sensitivity. Choose fresh food that has not been packaged or frozen so you can experience subtle, natural flavors.

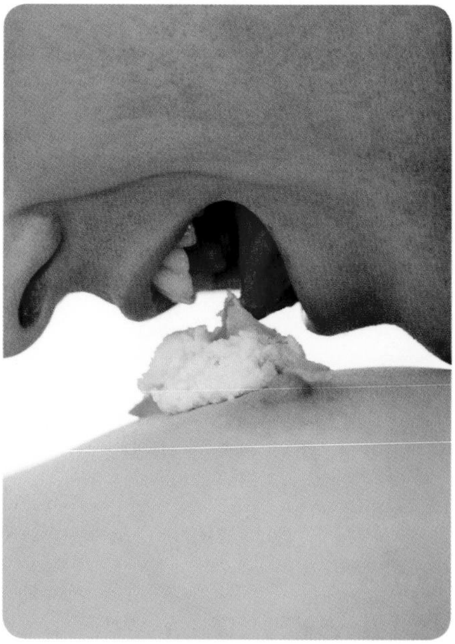

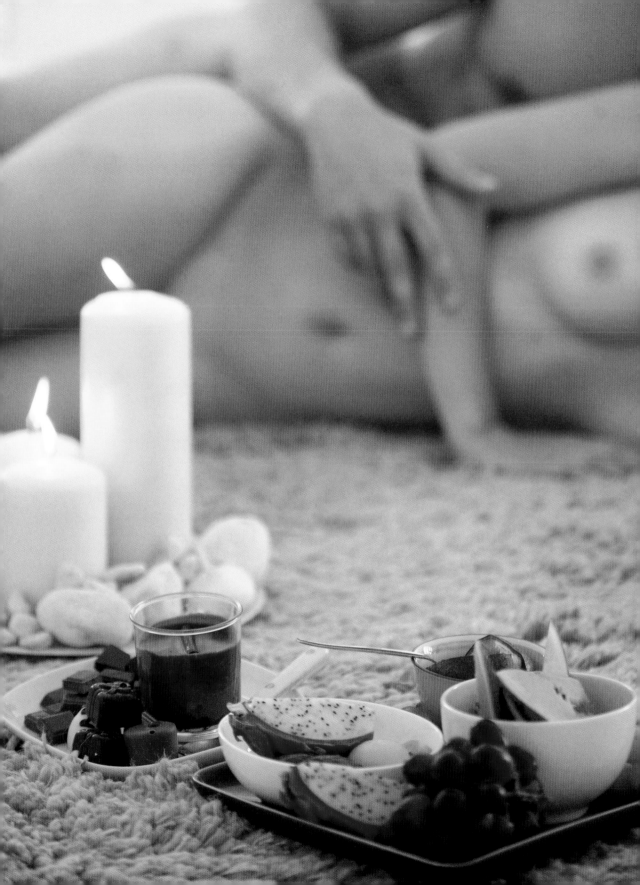

Sound

Tantra gives equal attention to each one of our senses, to bring the elements of life into balance. Becoming attuned to the subtleties of sound is an important part of that journey. A sexy whisper, an attractive voice, or a piece of music can all be potent aphrodisiacs.

chakra notes

Sound is vibrational energy that moves through matter in wave form. Different parts of the body vibrate at different oscillations, so it makes sense that certain notes will resonate with corresponding organs and chakras. For example, the base chakra resonates at the note of "C". The heart vibrates at the note of "F". There are healers that use singing bowls and tuning forks to stimulate and balance the body and the chakra system. When you are aware of this concept you can see why music affects us so profoundly on all levels, physically as well as emotionally.

rhythm and sex

Music with rhythm can serve as a provocative generator in lovemaking. Sex is rhythmic–whether it's slow and seductive or fiery and feral, with two bodies becoming synchronized in a subtle dance, flowing in and out of the beat. An atmospheric musical soundtrack can play a large part in creating the ambience during tantric sex, inspiring different moods such as playful, tender, wild, gentle, primal, and ecstatic. When you need some support in keeping the energy high during lovemaking, rhythmic music with a sexy beat is the ideal tool. Sound will ignite your body with an expansive energy, allowing it to follow its own innate and spontaneous motion.

sensual speech

A sensual voice with warm, cheeky undertones can also be a powerful turn-on, and can set the mood for physical and emotional intimacy. Make time to talk with, and really listen to your partner, and to notice each other's particular timbre and inflection. Notice how your voice becomes calm when you relax, and be aware of nuances of tone. You can generate feelings of great excitement with the way you say things; speak

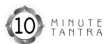

MINUTE TANTRA

OM VIBRATION

This simple and relaxing method is a way to bring unity and balance to a relationship. For Hindus and Buddhists, Om signifies the primordial sound, the first breath of creation, and the vibration that manifests existence.

- Namaste each other (see page 10).
- Sit opposite your partner. Breathe in deeply and chant the sound "Om" together. The emphasis should be on the "mmm."
- Let your two notes become one harmonious resonance. You should begin to feel your bodies vibrate. Don't force anything; allow the vibration to build as you chant.
- Namaste each other to finish.

☺ Read to each other

Reading sexy, erotic literature to one another makes great foreplay. There is an eclectic array of stimulating stories on the market these days. (See Resources, page 186.) Take turns reading to one another. Really get into the spirit of it, and use your sexiest voice. Linger on the words and bring the story to life with your vocal expression. Let humor play its part; laughter is also a great aphrodisiac.

calmly, sexily, or with excitement, and notice how you both respond. If you sound excited, your partner will pick up on your energy. During foreplay and while you make love, whisper loving, and rude and erotic sound-bites into your partner's ear. Sound can be a great sexual stimulant, and can help bring real focus to the moment. Hear him gasp when you describe a fantasy or suggest something you want him to do; feel her melt as you declare your passion straight from the heart.

SYMBOLIC OM

The symbol "Om" signifies the oneness of all creation. There is a belief, echoed throughout the world's faiths and traditions, that universal matter was created by sound. The sign for "Om" is the main symbol of the Hindu religion, placed at the start of the sacred texts.

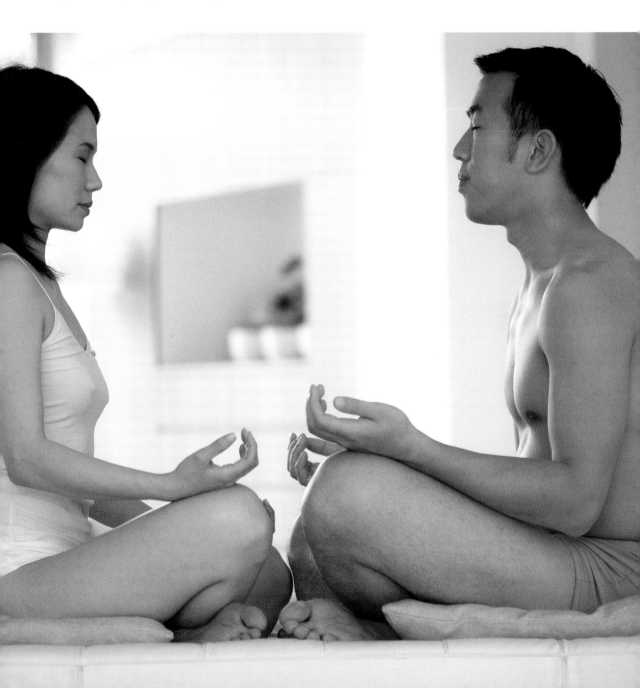

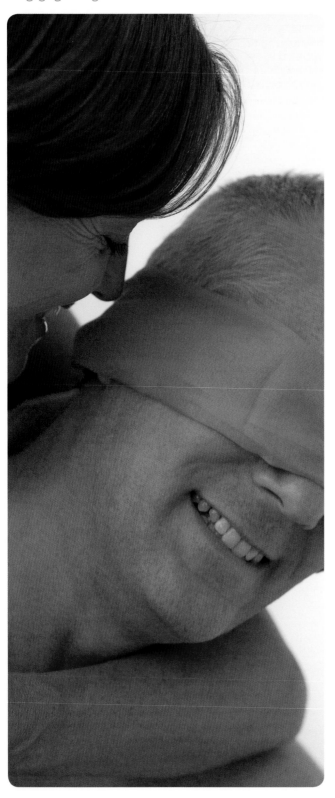

sharing music

Enjoying music with your beloved is a simple, yet profound way of journeying into bliss together. When you listen to music in the company of another person, it can enhance the experience, allowing the music to penetrate deep into your body. The mutual sharing of music can be an auditory adventure, creating a sense of ecstatic rapture on a cellular level.

1 Put on some slow and relaxing music that you both enjoy (see Resources, page 186).

2 Lie comfortably together and close your eyes. Listen without speaking. Disappear into the sound, letting thoughts drift away.

3 Let the music fill your body, touching your heart and soul. Relax in this musical bliss for at least 20 minutes.

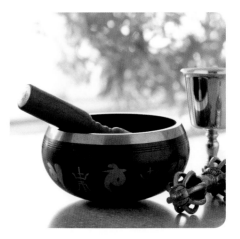

SINGING BOWL

This simple instrument is easy to play and produces an enchanting tone that has the power to transport the listener into altered states of consciousness.

opening to sound

In this meditation you sing for each other. You may giggle at first, especially if you're not used to singing in front of anyone else, but see if you can move beyond that, and get into the spirit of the meditation. Singing for a one-person audience is a truly intimate act, and can be a channel straight to the heart of your beloved.

1 Namaste each other (see page 10).

2 The man should sit or recline in a comfortable position. Blindfold him, so he can focus his senses on your voice.

3 Whisper words of love and devotion to him. Be spontaneous, and let the mood of the moment inspire you. Hum a gentle tune, like a mother singing to her child. This can be a profound healing experience for a man.

4 Play your singing bowl, and sing for five minutes.

5 After five minutes, switch roles and ask your partner to whisper and sing to you. Men, be generous with your whispered words of adoration. Reach down into the depths of your creativity. Let your words be both tender and erotic. Sing for your beloved—don't worry about what the song is. Even a nursery rhyme will be welcomed.

6 Play the singing bowl for five minutes. You can play it on its own, or sing or hum along with it.

7 Namaste each other to complete.

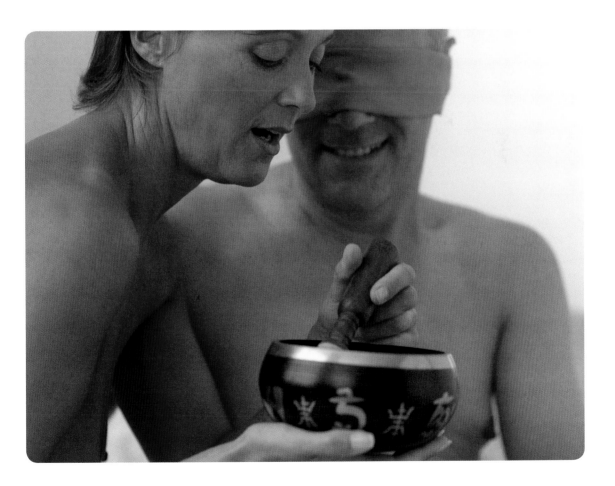

Touch

Touch is the sense related to the heart chakra. A caring touch brings nourishment to the body, mind, and soul, and can enhance a person's feeling of self-esteem and wellbeing. It also increases their sense of arousal and desire, and heightens anticipation for further contact.

sensual touch

Partners communicate their feelings for one another in a variety of ways, but there is nothing that transmits love as powerfully as touch. Both men and women truly blossom when they are touched with sensitivity, love, and consciousness.

The skin is the largest organ of the body, and connects us from top to toe. It also serves as the interface between our inner reality and the world around us. Hands and fingers contain some of the densest areas of nerve endings on the human body. When we touch another person, we are creating a powerful alchemy, sending complex sensual messages backward and forward between two bodies. Touch has the capacity to fuse together two bodies, creating the experience of a single breathing and feeling being. You can take this awareness into your tantric sexual relationship, as a conduit for shared bliss.

healing touch

As humans we are conduits for healing energy. You don't have to be a trained masseur or body worker in order to channel healing energy through your hands. You are born with that gift, and you choose whether to use it or not.

Miracles can happen for partners when they are willing to journey on the path of tantra together. Lovers can bring a deep healing to their beloved simply through purposeful, gentle touch. A caress is a way to show and experience love, and move into a timeless space, beyond the mind. Tantra also brings in the spiritual element through ritual, creating deep relaxation such as after lovemaking, and inspiring reverence for your partner, as a divine being whom you are honored to be touching.

receiving touch

This simple exercise can help to bring awareness to the subtle nuances of touch, and it is wonderful to receive mindful, loving touch. Aim to convey love through your hands; this can take a little practice, but consider the time you spend refining your ability to touch as a gift you can give to your partner.

1 Ask your partner to lay down on cushions, naked. Blindfold him to focus his other senses.

2 Blow gently across his body. If you have long hair, run it over his chest and belly.

3 Stroke feathers lightly over his skin. Touch parts of his body, tenderly. Caress his skin with your fingertips. Let your imagination have full rein. Experiment and touch parts of his body in ways you've never touched before. You can use your mouth, your tongue, and your feet.

4 Change around so it is the woman's turn to receive her partner's loving touch.

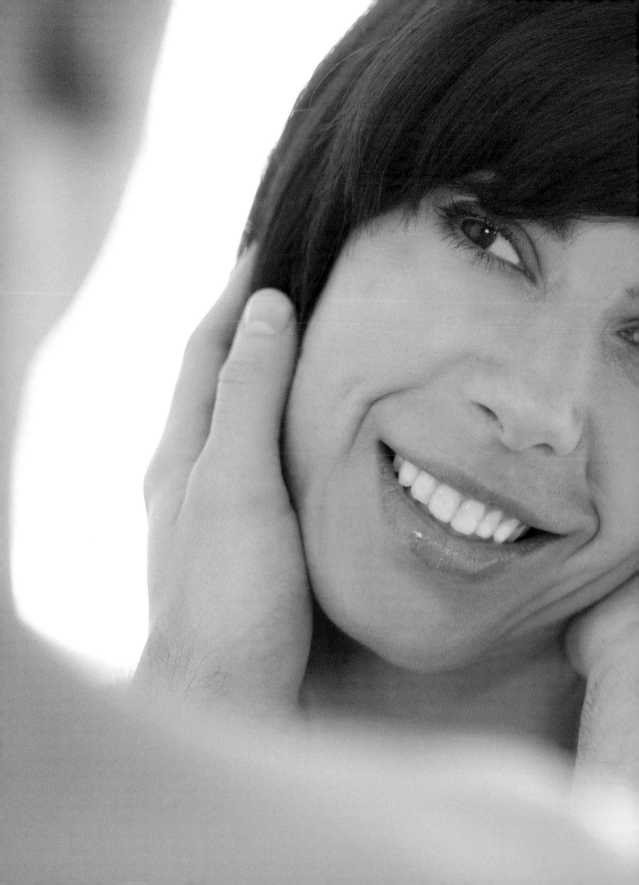

blindfold touch

This simple exercise can help to bring awareness to the subtle nuances of touch. Spending some time refining your sense of touch is a wonderful gift you can give to your partner. For this exercise, use items that have different feels. They could be soft, hard, cold, furry, wet, warm, metal, wood—anything will do. Practicing this meditation with sex toys can be a fun alternative.

1 Blindfold your partner.

2 Bring the first item to your partner's skin, choosing a spot that doesn't usually get much attention. Earlobes, cheeks, shoulders, and fingertips are all remarkably sensitive areas. Tease your partner with a fleeting touch, or press the object against the skin, creating patterns or shapes.

3 Choose the next item and repeat the meditation. Aim for a contrasting sensation to increase sensitivity—for example, follow up a light, teasing touch with a feather by rubbing an ice cube across the skin.

4 Swap places so the second partner can experience different types of touch.

☉ Buying tantric toys

Sex toys can enhance your love life and inspire imaginative and creative lovemaking. As you become more sensitive, you will probably find that you need less stimulation for arousal. For tantric sex, the more subtle the toy the better. Try experimenting with feathers, dildos made from glass or quartz crystal, Ben Wa balls and prostate massagers, which are all tactile in nature. Using these items to touch your partner in various ways and places can enrich and enliven your sexual playtime and further increase your sensitivity. Some people find spanking highly erotic. If you're looking for whips or paddles, it's worth buying ones made from high-quality materials.

If you're a Shakti waiting for your Shiva to come along, and you want to invest in a vibrator, there are some hi-tech versions on the market. Look especially for ones made with medical-grade silicon.

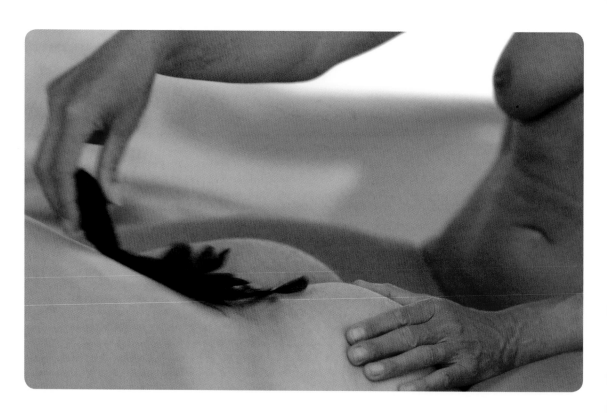

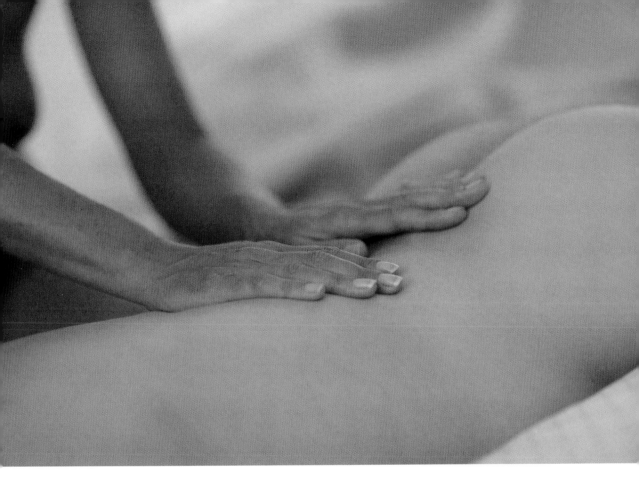

enter the caress

If done regularly, this meditation can have a healing effect on any sexual problems—such as premature ejaculation, impotence, or frigidity—by awakening sensitivity and stimulating pleasure throughout the entire body. Switch between acting as the giver and the receiver. Here, the man is the first to receive the caress.

1 Ask your partner to lie face down. Rest both hands lightly on his back and feel his breath rising and falling.

2 Caress his body with one hand, slowly and hypnotically. You are gently leading and traveling with your partner into a meditative state, a space beyond time and mind.

3 Keep your hand as flat as possible. Transmit love through the gentle movement of your hand. Take 10 minutes to lovingly caress the back of his body.

4 Ask your partner to turn over. Use your fingers to gently

caress his face. Move your hand continuously, and try to avoid jumping to different parts of the body. Every so often, softly whisper the sutra, "Enter the caress, sweet prince as everlasting life."

5 Enter a state of deep meditation together; you are not trying to arouse your partner.

6 After 10 minutes you can withdraw your hand and sit silently, allowing your partner to come back.

7 Change around, so the woman becomes the receiver.

chakra touch

This massage awakens the chakras (see page 20). Chakra massage is a joy to give, as well as to receive. As the giver, you can set your partner's chakras spinning with a simple, circular motion of your fingertips. You may choose to take it in turns to give and receive this massage, or you may choose to devote time to just one partner, as a loving, generous treat.

You will find the massage has stimulated the chakras, making them energized and alive. As a result, this meditation leads beautifully into lovemaking.

Before you start, make sure the room is warm, and you have a blanket within easy reach to cover your partner, if desired. Have your oils readily to hand. Warm your hands and the oils before you start. Choose an aromatic blend that energizes and stimulates your partner, rather than putting them to sleep!

1 The man lies down with a cushion under his head for comfort. He should be naked.

2 The woman puts oil onto her fingers. Slowly, and in a clockwise direction, apply the oil to his first chakra, located at the hairline on the pubic bone, for two to three minutes. After massaging each chakra point, always rest your hand there for a moment, and feel the energy rising.

3 Move on to his second chakra, located halfway between his navel and the pubic hairline. Reapply oil to your fingers between each chakra, and massage in a circular motion.

4 Move on to his third chakra, located halfway between his navel and the end of his sternum.

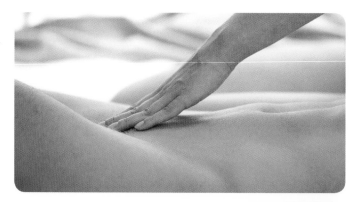

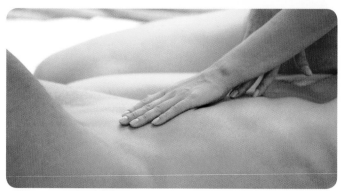

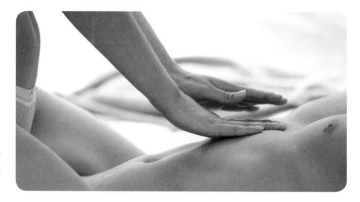

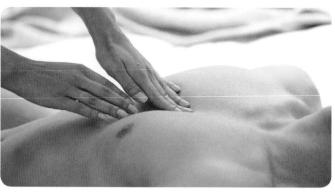

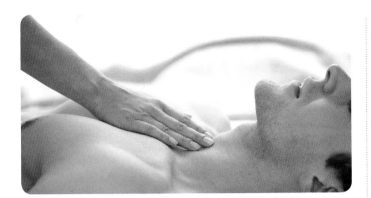

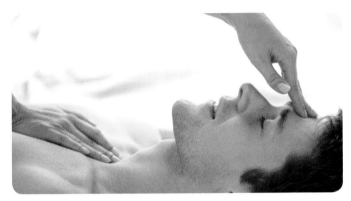

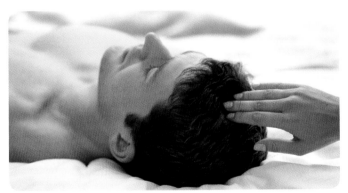

5 Move on to his fourth chakra, located at the center of his chest, between his nipples. This is the heart chakra, and it is especially intimate to give and receive touch here.

6 Move on to his fifth chakra, located below his Adam's apple. Use a light touch, especially when resting your hand.

7 Move on to his sixth chakra, located at the center of his forehead. Instead of circles, stroke upward from between his eyebrows to his hairline in a gentle sweeping motion.

8 Dry your fingers, as you don't need oil for the seventh chakra. Find his crown chakra by drawing an imaginary line from the top of his ears to the top of his head. Imagine the top of his head like a clock face, and slowly massage with two fingers in a clockwise direction, resting your hand there a while. This chakra connects your partner to the universe, and he should feel the energy of the universe entering him, merging with his own energy.

9 Place your hands gently, one on the base chakra and one on the crown. This connects heaven and earth, sex and spirit. It also brings the man's awareness to the flow of energy up and down the central channel of his body.

10 Give your partner a chance to relax and rest in quiet, energized bliss after the massage.

11 Change places so that the woman receives the massage, and then move into lovemaking, if you choose.

☾ Mixing your own massage oils

There are plenty of massage oils available to buy, but blending your own unique combination adds to the sense of ceremony and preparation before a tantric massage. Blending your own oils means that you can create something special that will truly appeal to your partner. Before you massage, offer the individual aromatherapy oils to your partner, and see which he or she responds to. To get started, try the following mixtures:

For the man: lemon, cedar, sandalwood, and patchouli

For the woman: rose, neroli, and jasmine

Sight

Sight is considered the most complex of the five main senses. It is the sense that gives us the most information about the world around us. Tantra focuses on the psychological aspect of seeing–that is, perception–as well as evoking the erotic possibilities.

tantric sight

Sexually speaking, it is clear that most people, and especially men, are very aroused by the way a partner, the object of desire, looks. Taking time to prepare to give your partner a stimulating visual experience can become not only part of the anticipation of union but also part of the devotional and meditative spiritual practice that is the coming together of Shiva and Shakti.

We respond deeply to being invited into a warm and sacred space that has been prepared by a lover. Imagine the sensual experience of soft candlelight, the musky aroma of incense and perfume, and carefully chosen music, with you sitting receptively at the center of this sacred space, prepared and beautiful. This visual feast will arouse your partner in a profoundly sacred way. With eyes wide open your partner will smile as he approaches you. He will embrace and kiss you with the love he feels written all over his face for you in turn to see.

yin yang vision

In tantra the aim is to drop judgments about what you see, and to diminish the amount of time you spend analyzing. Usually, we look at the world with "yang" vision. This is a masculine way of seeing–active, creative, and also opinionated. There's nothing wrong with this way of looking; it's simply that most people are unaware that there is another way of looking entirely– a "yin" vision. Yin vision is used during tantric meditations.

Yin vision is a softer, more receptive way of seeing, where you soften your gaze and receive through your eyes, like a gift. You don't even "use" your eyes as such; you are almost in a trance state. In this place of quiet acceptance, you can really see and perceive the heart of the person or object in front of you.

MANDALA

A powerful tool for enhancing one's vision, a mandala is a picture of geometric patterns that represent the cosmos, both symbolically and metaphysically. It depicts a microcosm of the universe from the human perspective.

Within every mandala (or *yantra*) is a central sacred circle. This reflects the circular form of your eye as you gaze at it during meditation. As your gaze relaxes and expands into the heart of the yantra, a spiritual stillness awaits. You will be using yin vision (see opposite).

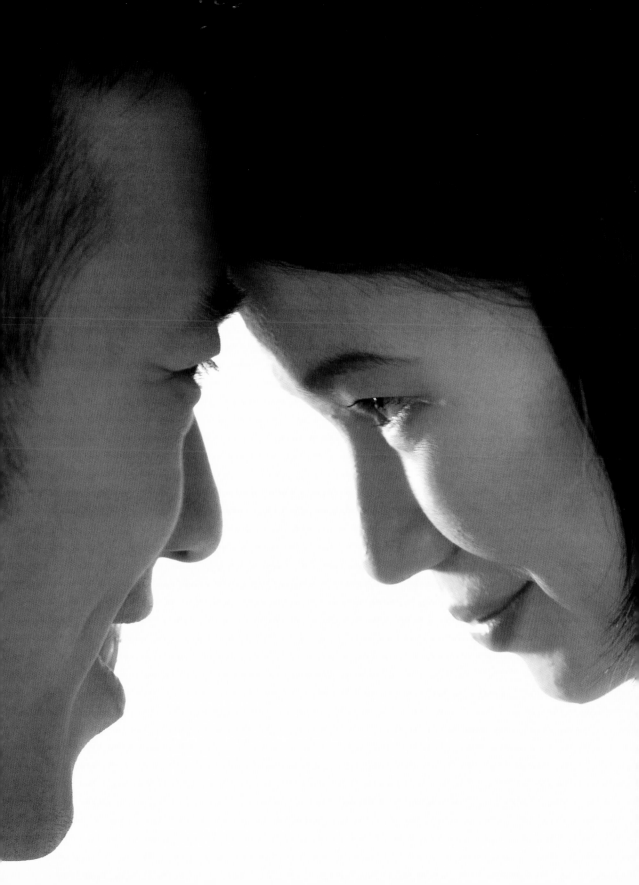

yin yang gazing

This is a beautiful meditation to perform before lovemaking. You can retain your yin vision while you make love. In doing so, you will allow your partner to expand into his or her full beauty and magnificence. Yin yang gazing is a way of seeing into the Buddha nature of each other—loving, quietly powerful, and infinitely wise.

1 Perform the opening ceremony (see page 12).

2 Sit opposite each other, as close as you can get with enough light to be able to see your partner's face clearly.

3 Let your eyes wander naturally across the face of your partner, taking in all the details of skin, colors, and features.

4 Look at your partner's hair, neck, and ears. Allow the movement of your eyes to be free and spontaneous.

5 Notice how your mind has something to say about almost everything your eyes fall upon. Don't try to hold onto these opinions—allow them to drift away as your gaze moves to the next feature, and let your thoughts follow their natural pattern without effort. Do this for five minutes. Notice how you see beauty, and how your partner transforms before you.

6 Close your eyes and rest for a few minutes.

7 Open your eyes again, and this time "soften" your eyes. Allow your partner to gaze into you. Receive his or her look, and let them penetrate you with their gaze. Concentrate on how it feels to be looked into in this intense way. Both partners are in fact "receiving" the intense gaze at the same time, but don't let this distract you.

8 After five minutes, close your eyes and rest again.

9 Open your eyes and let them rest upon a point somewhere between your two faces. You will probably find yourself sinking into a deeply meditative state. Rest in the peace for a few minutes until you become alert again.

10 Perform the closing ceremony (see page 12).

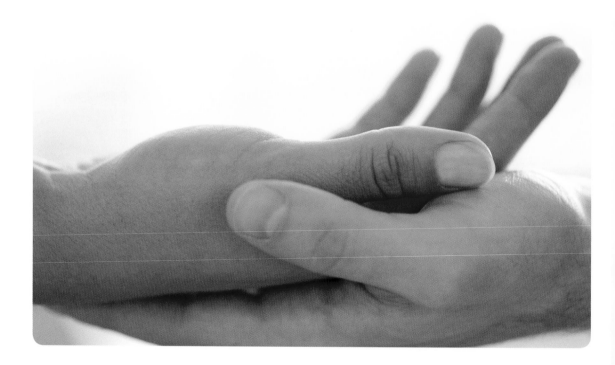

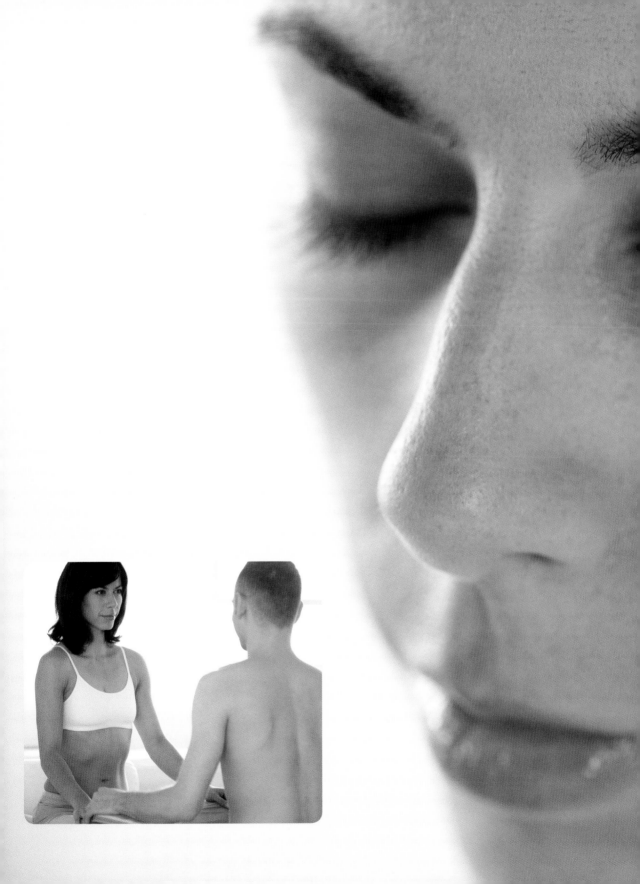

dancing the divine

In this meditation you dance to reveal your true nature, rather than to perform. When it is your turn to watch, soften your gaze and be receptive. Revel in the sight of your partner being so open and playful. When it is your turn to dance, relax and let your body lead your movements.

1 Namaste each other (see page 10).

2 Put on some gorgeous, sexy music that appeals to you both. The woman then sits or lies on a sofa or cushions.

3 The man begins to dance, slowly removing each item of his clothing. Take your time over every layer, looking your partner in the eye as much as possible.

4 The woman should not make any comments. Simply receive the scene using yin vision (see page 108). Welcome your sexy partner into your heart and soul.

5 When you have stripped to become fully naked, dance to celebrate your freedom and sexuality, moving to express every aspect of your inner divine essence.

6 Change places so the man is watching and the woman is stripping and dancing for her partner. Give him your full attention. If you feel embarrassment, let that be there, incorporate it into your dance; it will soon shift and dissipate.

7 At the end, dance together, enjoying each other's beauty.

8 Namaste each other to finish.

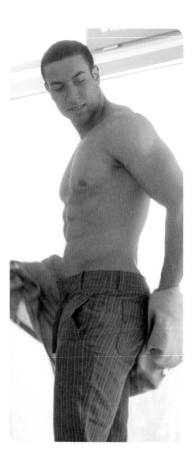
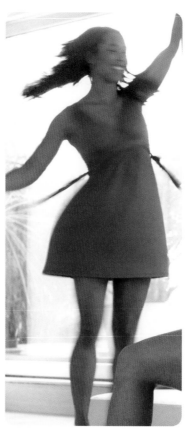
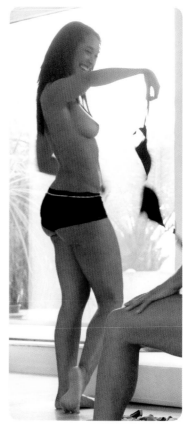

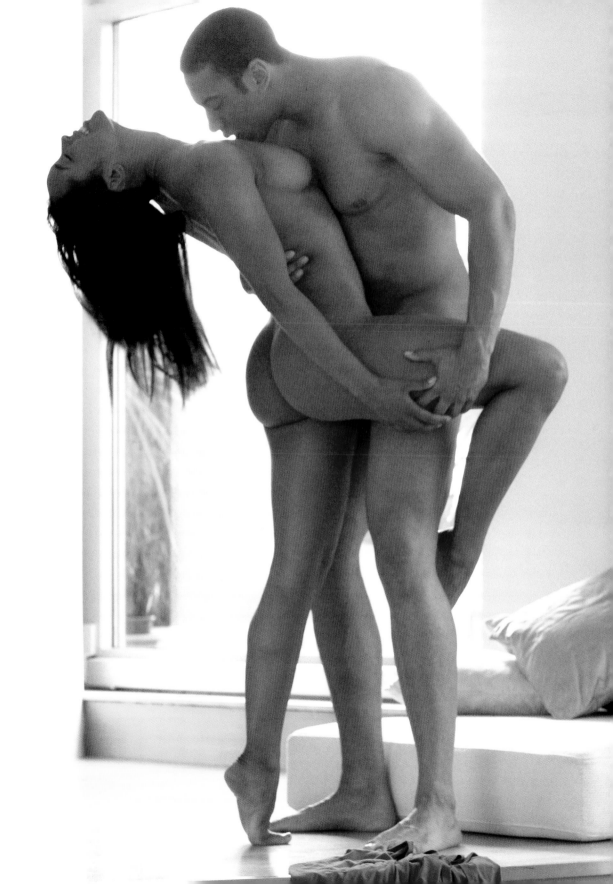

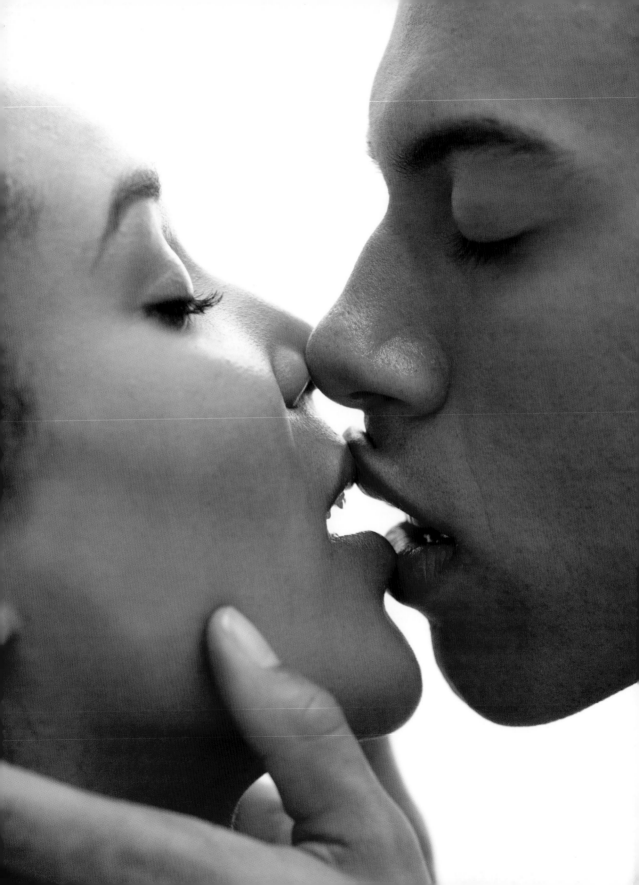

7

ENGAGE WITH YOUR BODIES

In tantra we encourage you to engage with your partner with every part of your body. Breathing, kissing, massaging—each one of these simple activities can create a magical, deeply sensual experience. The way to get there is to dwell in your bodies fully, stay in tune with your partner, and to dive deeply into each erotic moment, letting everything else fall away.

Breath

In tantra, breath is considered the single most powerful tool for transformation. The deeper you breathe, the more you feel, and tantra encourages you to feel everything to its full potential. Deep, relaxed breathing will energize you completely, filling you with vitality.

breath and the body

In tantra, breath is considered the gateway to the divine. If you breathe in a thoughtful way, energy will follow the flow of that breath, bringing fresh energy in its wake. As you fill with energy and vitality, your senses will heighten, and you will be more open to receiving divine pleasure.

As you grow more aware of your breath and how it affects you, you will gain a greater understanding of your body. You will relax more, bringing an enhanced confidence and creativity to each moment. If you feel under pressure, use breath to calm yourself. Make time to get outside on a daily basis, to walk and breathe in the fresh air, and expel the stale air. You will be more able to access realms of subtle energy, especially during sex.

breath and sex

Tantra encourages deep breathing to activate all the areas of the body. When you breathe in, you flood your body with fresh oxygen, which enlivens every cell and makes you feel alive and energized. This is the gateway to experiencing a full body orgasm, where every part of your body, not just your genitals, is alive with sensation and pleasurable feelings. By breathing deeply during massage, foreplay, and sex you encourage the feelings of enjoyment you experience to flow all around your body. If you hold your breath you will restrict your pleasure and emotional release. The more you breathe, the more pleasurable feelings will move about your body.

breathing together

Breathing with your partner is an important part of many tantric meditations, and can help harmonize your two beings. It helps you to relax and bring your attention to each other. When

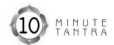

MINUTE TANTRA

WAKE UP YOUR BODY

When you breathe through your chakras, they wake up and begin to spin more actively. This allows your whole body to fill with vitality. In turn this leads to a more active, pleasure-filled, and vibrant sex life. Do this breathing meditation whenever you need to energize your body. It is especially effective outdoors.

1 Sit quietly and focus on your breath. Notice how it rises and falls as you breathe in and out. Be aware of the point where it turns around at the top of the in breath and falls back down again on the out breath.

2 Bring your attention to your stomach. As you inhale and exhale with long slow breaths, keep your awareness on your stomach. On each out breath, let any tensions held in the belly float away. Imagine the breath carrying the stress out of your body. Gradually you will feel more relaxed as your muscles loosen up.

3 Now imagine that you're receiving a breath in through your base chakra. Breathe up into your second chakra, then breathe out back down to your base. Continue to breathe in this way, creating a loop of energy between your first and second chakras. Continue for about 15 minutes, then return to regular breathing.

you breathe together, you become one, becoming fully aware of the moment you share together. This cosmic union is the ultimate goal of tantric lovers.

Before and during tantric lovemaking, use the conscious breathing methods explained on the next four pages. These are designed to help you to learn to control your breathing. As you breathe, your bodies will calm down and help you to leave the worries of the day behind. Oxygen will flood your bodies, making them feel energized and enlivened. Your muscles will relax and your senses will become more alert. You will find that you are mentally and physically more alert for lovemaking.

HOW BREATH IMPACTS ORGASM

Breathing deeply can stimulate a strong sexual charge, enhancing your body's orgasmic potential. Breath is also the key to being able to let go and surrender to the joy of the moment. As you orgasm, breathe out, to let the orgasmic energy flow throughout your whole body. In some meditations, it is suggested that you tense your body. Try holding your breath, before breathing out and releasing, which enhances the feeling of release when you finally let go.

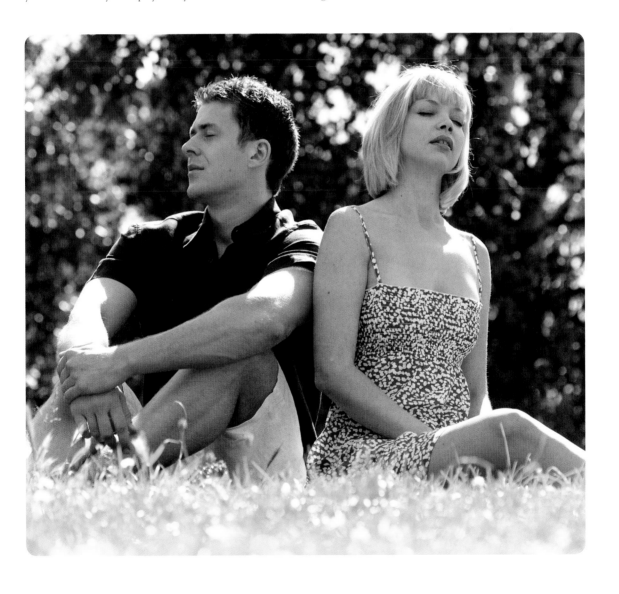

circular breathing

This breathing meditation helps to align the chakras between two partners, clearing any blockages that may inhibit the natural flow of sexual energy. As you breathe together you will find the rhythm of your bodies synchronizes. Your pulse rates will calm, and you will feel fully relaxed. You don't need to force your breath—take your time, relax your mind, and a miraculous harmonization will occur.

1 Perform the opening ceremony (see page 12).

2 Sit opposite each other on a bed or sofa, or on a comfortable rug. Rest your hands on your knees.

3 Breathe in and out slowly, taking long, deep breaths. Keep your eyes open to start with so that you can watch your partner. Do this for five minutes, with an unforced rhythm.

4 Change the pace of your breaths so that when the man breathes out, the woman breathes in. Do this for five minutes so you establish a relaxed rhythm together.

5 The woman imagines that she is breathing in through her first chakra (from the base of her body) and taking the breath up through her body to her heart chakra. She then breathes out from her heart chakra and back down the front of her body.

6 At the same time, the man imagines breathing in through his heart chakra, taking the breath down through his body and sending it out from his base chakra. Imagine that the two breaths create a circle between the man and the woman. Breathe in this relaxed way for five minutes.

7 Change around, so that the woman is breathing out from her base chakra, and the man is breathing out from his heart chakra. Continue for five minutes.

8 Lie down in the star position, the man lying on his back, arms and legs outstretched. The woman lies between his legs, with her legs over his thighs. Allow your hands to touch the feet of your partner. Rest in this position, with easy breathing, for 10 minutes. Your bodies will be flooded with fresh oxygen, your chakras will spin, and every part of you will feel energized.

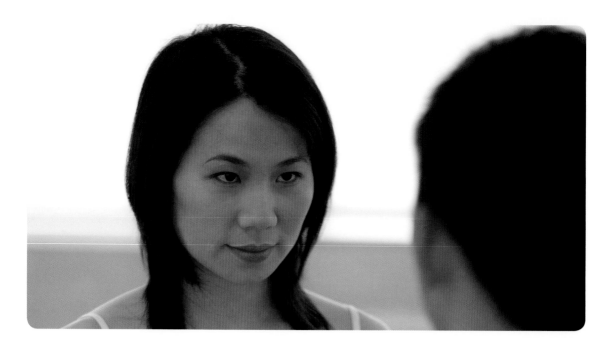

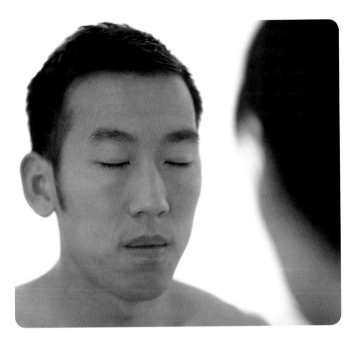

ᱰ Breathing during penetration

Circular breathing is sensual and unifying, and can be practiced during sex to heighten the sensations of penetration and orgasm.

During penetration, the man should visualize breathing out of his base chakra and lingam, and the woman should visualize breathing in through her base chakra and yoni. The man should keep his physical movements soft, and allow his body to effortlessly ride the waves of energy, keeping his attention on the circular breath he shares with his partner. The woman lets her breath bring deep release, receiving her partner to the very core of her being. As the woman breathes out, she relaxes her yoni to receive her partner fully.

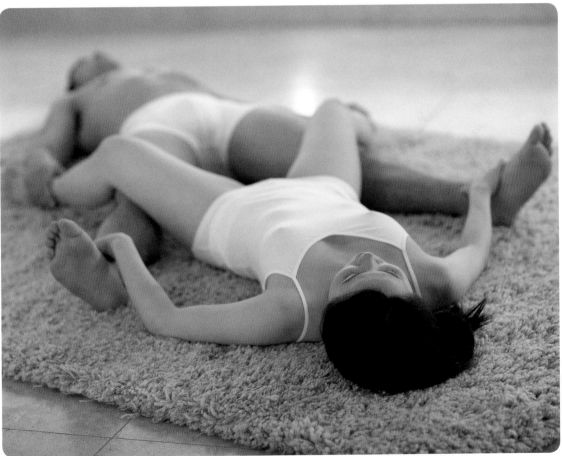

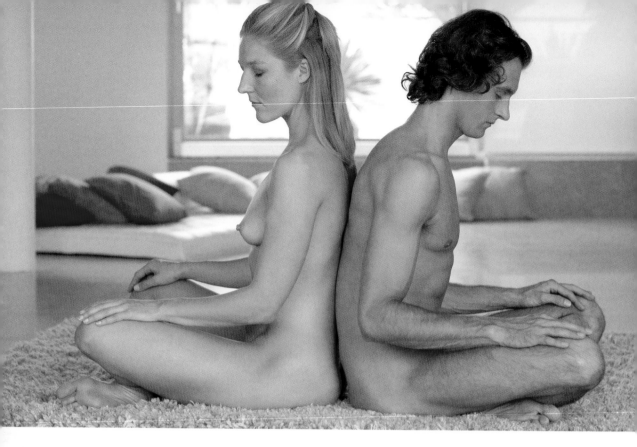

chakra breathing

This is a dynamic meditation that involves energetic breath, as well as vigorous, spontaneous, physical movement. It serves to expand your lung capacity, and also energizes every one of your chakras. If your relationship feels stagnant, this can help clear the path to increased energy, fluidity, and aliveness between you.

1 Perform the opening ceremony (see page 12).

2 Sit comfortably back to back. Both breathe in and out with an open mouth, directing your breath into your first chakra (at the base of your body). Allow your breath to be chaotic, sometimes slow and sometimes fast, making rough sounds as you exhale, like a panting dog.

3 Move your body as you breathe; let it shake or tremble or sway from side to side. Be careful not to bounce backward onto your partner's spine. Do this for one or two minutes.

4 Direct your breath into your second chakra (near your abdomen), and move as before. As the chakra is shaken open with the breathing and movement, let any emotions come to the surface and be expressed. Let out any sounds that may arise, whether a shout, cough, or laughter, and keep the breathing going throughout.

5 Continue to work your way up your chakras until you reach your crown chakra. Working from your base chakra to your crown chakra should take about 10 minutes.

6 Breathe back down through each chakra, allowing about 30 seconds for each. Your breath may start to calm.

7 Embrace for 15 minutes, feeling all of your chakras vibrating in unison. You may want to move into lovemaking after this meditation, enjoying the energy and intimacy that has been generated between you.

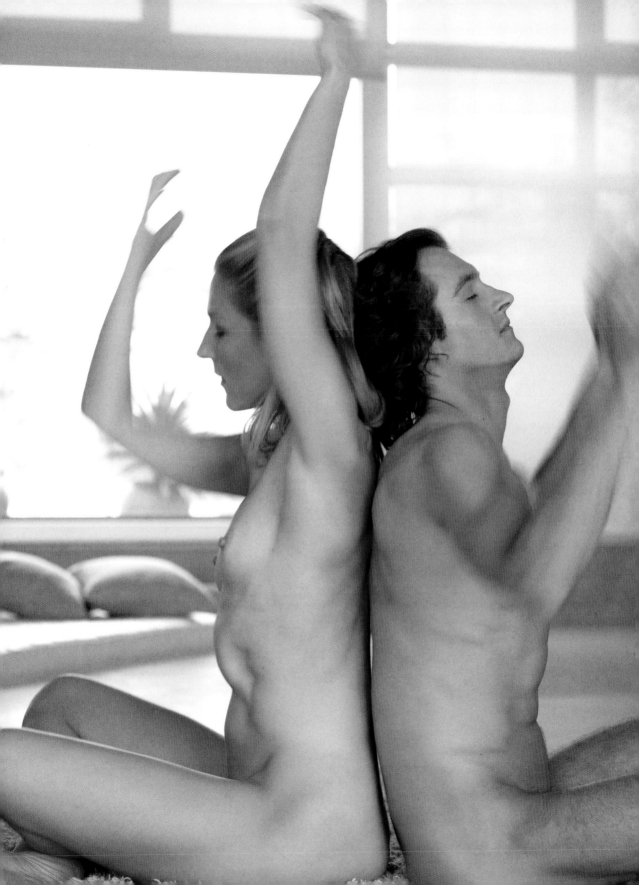

Kissing

Kissing is an intimate act that plays a crucial part in a couple's sex life. In order to have a passionate sex life, you need to be good at kissing. Kissing conveys your feelings, generates intimacy and energy, and sends subtle, sensual messages to your partner.

the importance of kissing

People connect romantically in a variety of ways, but the kiss, particularly the first kiss, can be a pivotal moment. It tells you right away if there is chemistry between you, and gives you a quick insight into whether you want to pursue this relationship. In a long-term relationship, kissing is an essential way to express your love and passion, and remind you that you are first and foremost lovers, whatever is going on in the world around you.

A kiss is also an important way to stimulate sexual compatibility between partners. The more you kiss, the more likely you are to be comfortable with each other. You are also more likely to be in tune with how your partner is feeling, and to know intuitively what type of physical contact he or she desires in that moment. And of course, good kissing is a perfect way to get you both in the mood for great sex.

the tantric kiss

Kissing mirrors the divine sexual union of Shiva and Shakti. It can be an intensely sexual experience–the sensual yielding of the lips is like the softness of the yoni and the penetrative tongue feels like the penetration of the lingam. In tantric sex, kissing plays an important role. Kissing sends erotic messages throughout the whole body, igniting flames of passion. A good kiss can heighten your senses, and plays a vital role in preparing you for tantric meditation and sex. The tantric kiss can be soft and tender or passionate and animalistic, but what makes it tantric is the focus and consciousness that you bring to it. Be aware of how you kiss, and how you feel when being kissed. This will increase your sensitivity to other parts of lovemaking.

☙ Kissing techniques

If you find you kiss in the same tried-and-tested way all the time, try some of these kissing techniques to see whether you can expand your repertoire. Choose ones which appeal to you both, and vary the order in which you try them, responding to your partner and the mood of the moment.

- Make eye contact with a soft gaze. Bring your lips together and brush lightly over the surface of each other's mouths, feeling your breaths meeting and merging. Lightly explore the surface of each other's lips.
- Let your tongue gently probe your partner's mouth and slowly twirl around the tip of his or her tongue. Keep your tongue relaxed. If you salivate too much during the kiss, pause for a while, then resume.
- Gently pull your partner's lower lip with your teeth, biting or sucking softly and tenderly. This can feel very sexy indeed.
- Try sucking your partner's tongue gently; this can feel very sensual.
- Kiss the back of your partner's neck and bite the top of his or her spine. Hold for a few seconds to give your partner a sudden rush of pleasure through their body.

initiating sex with kissing

The woman is considered the initiatress in tantra. This is because women possess the ultimate creative power–they can give birth to life. For women, kissing is especially significant because it triggers arousal and intimacy. The subtle clues that women get during a kiss are used as a means of monitoring the status of the relationship and measuring the commitment of their partner.

As a result, a woman may choose a lover based on how he kisses and whether a sexual relationship develops or not. Eighty five percent of women wouldn't consider intercourse without kissing. Statistically, most men consider kissing as a means to an end, and initiate kissing hoping that it will lead to sex. Knowing this about your partner should help to improve understanding on both sides. A male's saliva contains measurable amounts of testosterone that can affect the libido of his partner, another reason why kissing can turn on your partner.

A PHYSICAL REACTION

When two people kiss there is a complex exchange of chemical and tactile information. Both partners release hormones that make you feel sensual, relaxed, and alert, and which lead to sexual arousal. These hormones include measurable amounts of dopamine, endorphin, and phenylethylamine, feel-good hormones produced by the pituitary and hypothalamus glands. Endorphin hormones are natural opiates that bring a profound sense of wellbeing to a person, helping you move closer to a state of bliss and increasing your likelihood of orgasm.

Foreplay tends to include kissing, and for good reason. There is no better way to gauge the mood of your partner, and to arouse your bodies ready for physical contact.

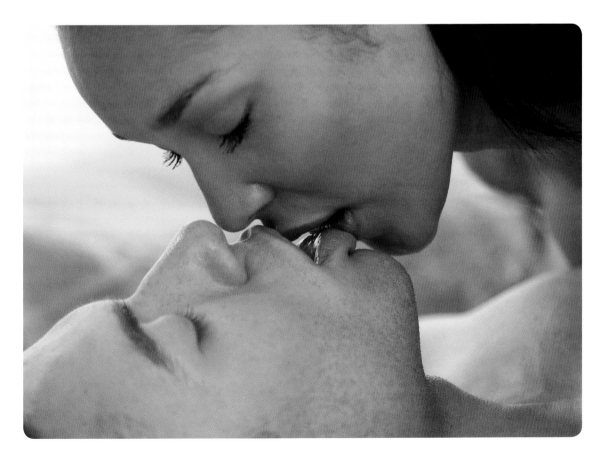

kiss exploration

This is a really romantic, sexy kissing meditation designed to bring back the memories of your first kiss together. You will bring into focus every desire, movement, and breath that occurs when kissing for the first time. To start, put on some slow and hypnotic background music that appeals to you both.

1 Stand as far away from each other as possible. Gaze at each other from afar for about five minutes. Be aware of your rising desire for contact and emotional connection.

2 Slowly, walk toward each other, step-by-step, looking into each other's eyes. Take as long as you can to reach each other.

3 When you meet, stand close without touching for five minutes. Look at your partner using yin vision (see page 108), softening your gaze and see the real person in front of you, rather than studying his or her features.

4 Gradually bring your mouths together and kiss as if for the first time. Taste, feel, and experiment with your lips and tongues.

5 After a few minutes pull apart slowly. While still looking into each other's eyes, move away from each other, walking backward. Notice how you feel when leaving your partner. As you separate, various emotions will arise, such as desire, loss, or grieving. Allow those emotions to be fully present in your body.

6 You may choose to move on to another meditation or to lovemaking, or simply sit and relax together, depending on how you feel.

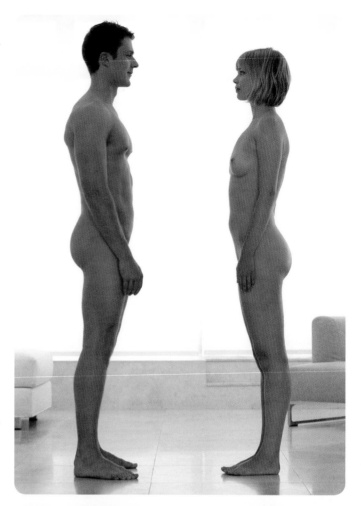

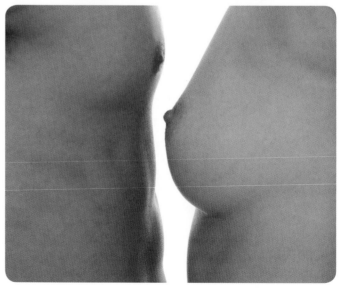

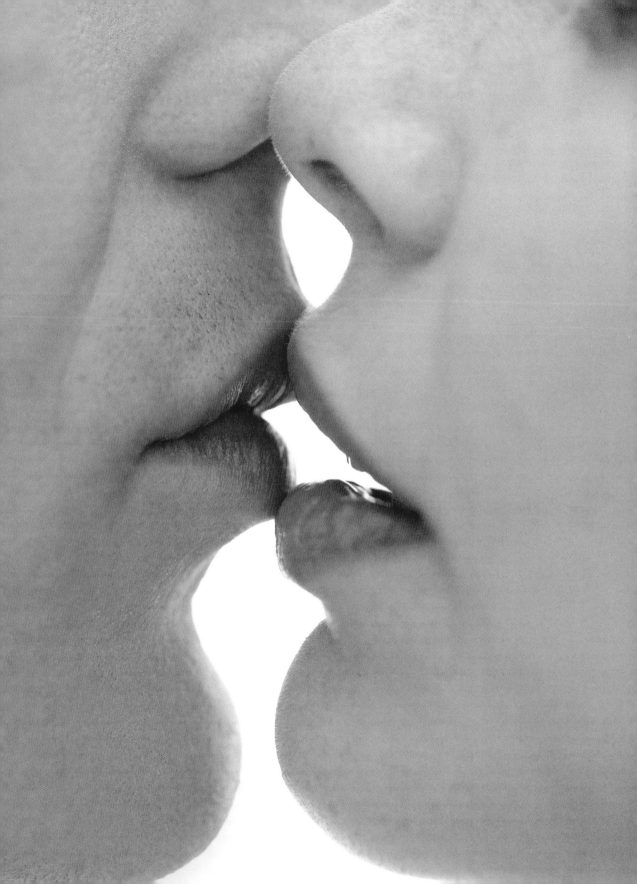

Erotic massage

Tantric massage can be used as a delicious form of foreplay that leads naturally into lovemaking. It is also a wonderful way to honor your partner's body. Massage provides both physical and emotional pleasure and can help to engender a deep level of trust between you.

awakening sexual energy

Erotic massage offers an excellent opportunity to practice communicating your sexual needs and likes to your partner. Partners can feel inhibited about speaking out loud their desires during penetrative sex, but during massage you can discover and explain what you like. You can massage when either of you wants to relax, even if you don't feel as if you would like to move into lovemaking. It can help to generate intimacy and dissolve stress. Massage can also be the starting point for an evening or weekend set aside for tantric meditation.

The sex energy generated during massage streams through your body and can transport both giver and receiver into a state of relaxed, deep meditation. As you both focus on your bodies, you will find that you cut out any mind-chatter, and the concerns of the day float away. When your mind has slowed down to a point where it becomes focused solely on the present, your body becomes balanced, receptive, and subtly rhythmic. This surrendered state is known in tantra as bliss.

becoming multi-orgasmic

Tantric massage is a great way to enhance and expand your sexual feeling. The path to becoming multi-orgasmic is to explore and heighten awareness of pleasure in every area of your body and your partner's body, not only the genitals.

Your skin is the largest sex organ of your body, so it deserves close attention. Massage the fingers, toes, the backs of your knees, ankles, neck, earlobes, and the crown of the head; all are erogenous zones known to generate sexual charge. As you lick, suck, caress, and massage you will both become open to the more subtle sensations of arousal. Your minds will relax and

---

MIXING MASSAGE OIL

The effects of your erotic massage can be greatly enhanced with the use of essential oils. I suggest you try the following recipe for a tantric massage oil. It is designed to stimulate and enhance feelings of love, sensuality, and relaxation:

- 8.5oz (250ml) jojoba, almond, or sunflower oil as a base oil
- 6 drops rose absolute
- 4 drops sandalwood
- 5 drops frankincense

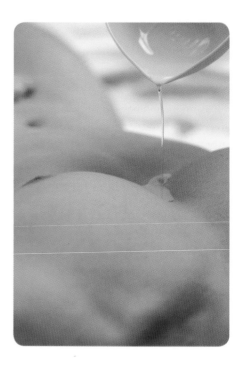

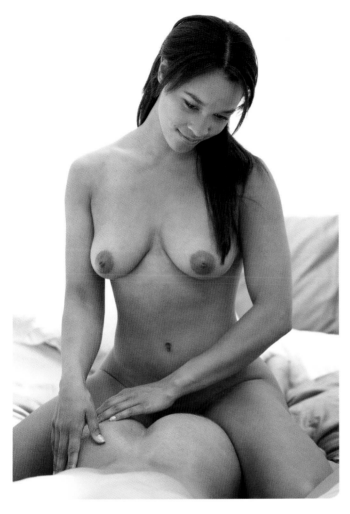

✆ Tips for erotic massage

Erotic massage is sexy and energizing, and can be as much fun to give as to receive. Technique is useful, but the most important thing is to bring conscious awareness and love to your massage. Here are some tips to make the massage easier and more comfortable for both of you:

- Massage your partner on a firm bed, or the floor, covering it with towels or sheets to protect it from massage oil.
- Make sure your hands are clean and your fingernails are short and smooth. Remove any jewelry before you start.
- Use an oil suitable for massage and that suits your partner. Check for allergies before use. If doing genital massage, use an appropriate lubricant. Check that it is compatible with condom use, if necessary.
- Warm the oil in your hands before applying it to the skin, by rubbing your hands together. Be liberal with the oil; it feels more sensual when your hands glide smoothly over the skin.
- Be confident; most massage moves feel great if given with love and consciousness. Think about each move, and repeat it to establish a comfortable rhythm.
- Be creative and don't be afraid to create new moves yourself. There are no mistakes in massage, as long as you remain aware of what you are doing.
- Don't massage your partner if he or she has undergone recent surgery, has heart problems, thrombosis, acute pain, contagious illness, or skin infection. If in doubt, seek medical advice.

focus on the moment. Take your time, and allow divine energy to enter and arouse your bodies. Use different types of touch to arouse varying sensations and lead to maximum arousal.

Tantric meditation is always connected with feelings of love and devotion. When you massage your partner, you will activate feelings of love within his or her heart chakra, creating a state of meditative bliss in preparation for a sublime orgasmic experience.

Tantric massage uses a calm, steady rhythm which builds and expands in gentle waves, reaching all parts of your body. You will find that your breath patterns begin to match the rhythm of the massage. As this rhythm builds within you, your body is more receptive to experiencing a full-body orgasm—one that can move throughout your body in waves.

erotic massage strokes

Try some of these ideas for erotic massage, and feel free to create your own. Experiment to see which you like to give and which your partner likes to receive. Make sure you honor the whole of your partner's body—don't just focus on the erogenous zones that you know will excite them. Allow your partner to relax and enjoy the massage, to engender a profound sense of trust.

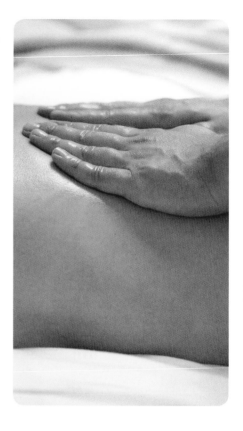

1 Flowing: long, sensuous strokes done with the whole hand or fingertips. Use plenty of oil so your movement flows with ease.

2 Kneading: rhythmic squeezing and releasing done by both hands pulling up large areas of skin. Use this on the more fleshy parts of the body such as the thighs, belly, hips, and buttocks.

3 Thumbing circles: small, deep movements using your thumbs. When done with pressure, this is a great stroke for releasing any tension held in the muscles, especially on fleshier parts of the body.

4 Feathering: light strokes using your fingertips. This delicate stroke stimulates the skin's sensory nerves, and makes the skin tingle.

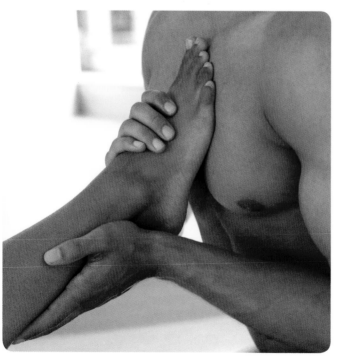

✆ Foot massage

Ritualized bathing and massaging of the feet has always been associated with devotional worship. On a subtle energy level, it is said that our feet are connected to karma and by massaging your partner's feet, you can heal emotional wounds incurred through negative events from the past.

On a physical level, every nerve in the foot connects with a nerve in the body. Consequently, your feet are highly sensitive, and massaging them sends pleasure signals throughout the entire body. A thorough foot massage can feel deeply relaxing and calming, with benefits for the whole body. If your partner's feet are ticklish, hold them firmly and massage more with your whole hand and less with your fingertips. It is possible to conquer ticklishness in the feet by regularly receiving massages.

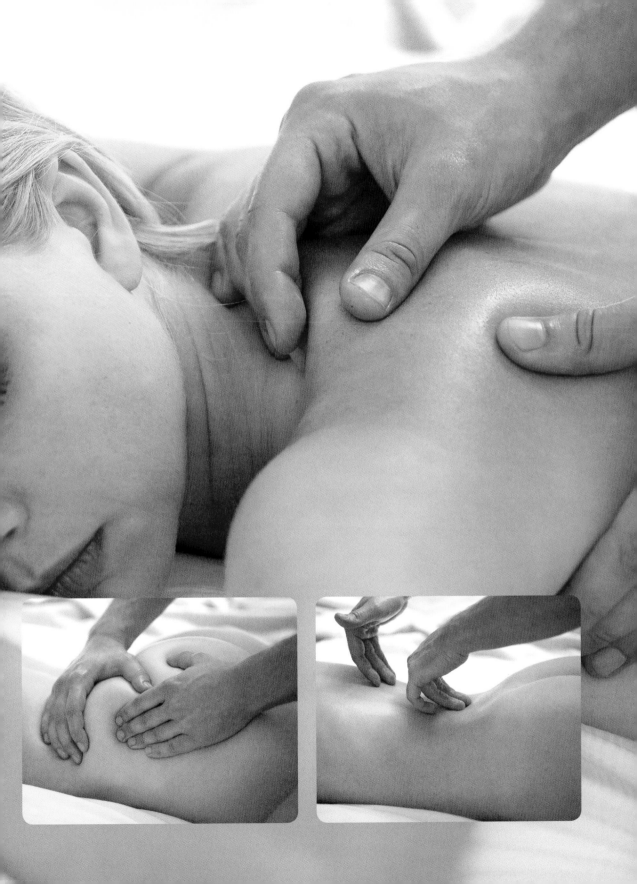

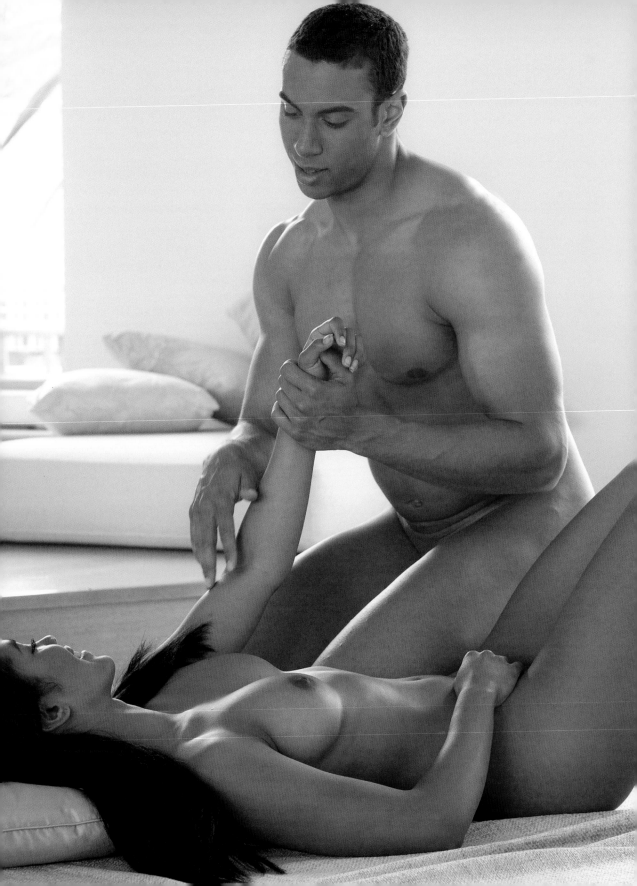

the touch game

It's important to find new ways to arouse your partner—and watching him or her enjoy your attention is very erotic for you, too. Take time to verbalize what turns you on or off. In this massage you will learn about your partner's likes and dislikes, and will also be able to share erotic secrets about yourself.

1 Get comfortable on a bed or rug, with one of you lying down. Using massage oil, start to massage your partner with simple strokes, such as a caress on the arm or leg.

2 Ask your partner as you massage, "How does this feel?"

3 If you are receiving the massage, be honest with your responses. Try to respond in a loving, constructive way, for example, "It feels great, but it might be even better if it were a little firmer," or, "It's a little ticklish just there. Could you try with the flat of your hand?" Massage for 5–10 minutes.

4 Change over. If you like, change again, and this time take some risks and invent new strokes.

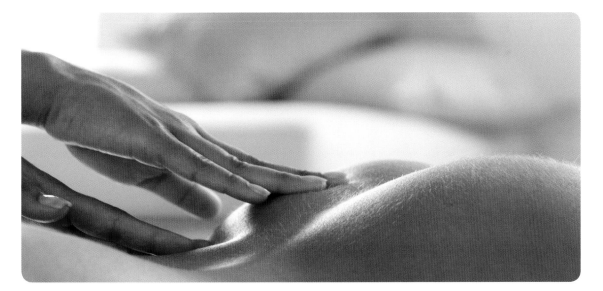

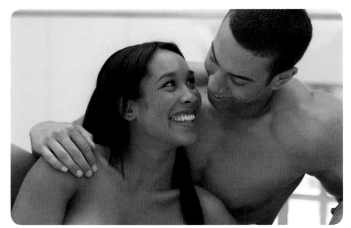

☜ Establishing boundaries

It is useful to have a short conversation outlining some rules and boundaries before you start your massage. These boundaries will allow the giver to feel confident and experiment within the massage, and they will allow the receiver to surrender fully while being massaged. You could agree which areas to miss out this time, or agree to give vocal feedback or stay silent throughout. You can state that you would rather sexual stimulation wasn't part of your massage.

lingam massage

To worship the lingam is to worship the man. A compassionate Shakti can bring her partner to a heightened awareness of his body's capacity for orgasmic pleasure through this massage. Perform this massage with patience and love, using firm but gentle strokes. Follow the sequence given, or vary it to respond to your partner's likes.

1 Start by massaging your partner's back, shoulders, and arms, then move down to his legs. Ask him to turn over, and massage his chest and thighs to encourage him to relax.

2 Using plenty of massage oil, cover his lingam, testicles, and perineum (located between the scrotum and the anus).

3 Using both hands, take long strokes to massage his lingam upward toward his chest, then move it gently out to the side, continuing to massage. Then bring his lingam down toward you, then to the other side, continuing to massage. Move his lingam clockwise slowly, massaging using a gliding motion.

4 Place both hands across his lingam and firmly pull them apart, stretching his lingam out lengthways. When your lower hand reaches his testicles, use your upper hand to hold his lingam in place against his body. Repeat a few times.

5 Use two fingers to massage his perineum in a circular movement. Place the middle finger of your other hand on the center of his forehead. Using firm pressure, press in to the perineum and stroke upward between his eyebrows up to the hairline. Remind him to breathe deeply throughout.

6 Slide your cupped hands in a rhythmic motion, one after the other down the shaft of his lingam. As one hand reaches the base, bring the other to the top and down again, in a continuous movement, so that the head of his lingam remains covered by your hands throughout.

7 Use both hands to rub the shaft of the lingam, sliding them around in opposite directions at the same time, as if you were wringing out a cloth. Repeat about 10 times.

8 Bring your hands, one after the other, down the shaft of his lingam 10 times. Then stop for a few seconds, holding his lingam firmly in both hands. Repeat, but count down nine strokes, then hold firmly. Continue until you reach one. If your partner feels like ejaculating, just stop and wait, then resume.

9 Finally, ask your partner to breathe in as deeply as he can, tensing his body for 20 seconds, before relaxing completely: the energy you have created will cascade through him.

☉ Discovering full-body orgasm

When there is no pressure for the man to perform as a lover, and his focus is taken away from ejaculation being the end result, his sexual energy can be directed into a full-body orgasm. Tense and release your muscles at the end of this massage, and your body will be overwhelmed with orgasmic energy, filling you with ecstatic pleasure.

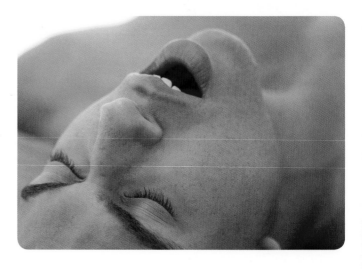

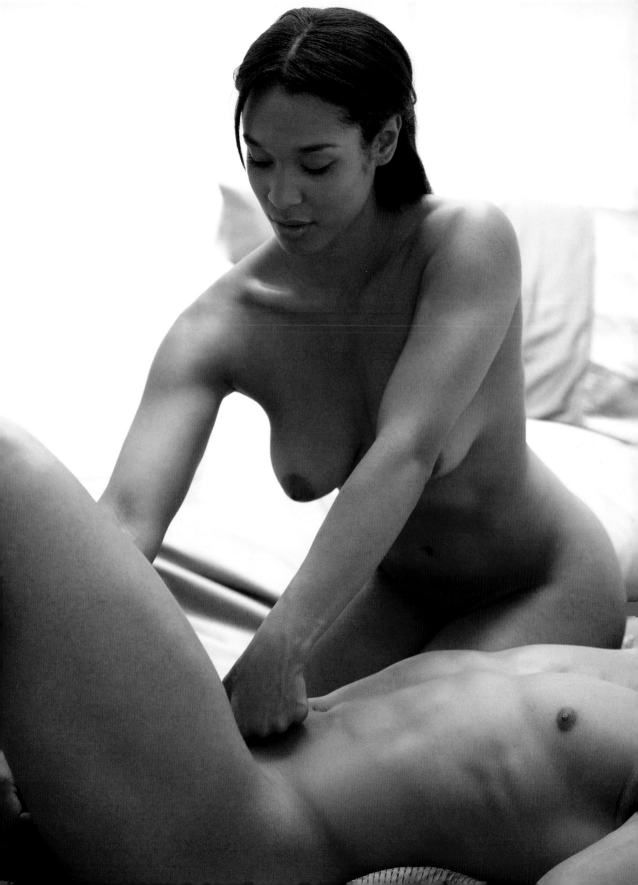

yoni massage

Receiving a yoni massage, where the partner has no agenda and is giving purely for the sake of your pleasure, is the ultimate gift for a woman. If the man is able to let go of any expectations around penetrative sex being the goal, the woman can relax fully, experiencing massage as a pure honoring of her goddess self. This helps her to surrender into tantric rapture, experiencing ecstatic bliss.

1 Begin by massaging your partner's shoulders, neck, and body, for as much time as you have, and allow your partner to relax completely. Remind her to breathe throughout.

2 Rest one hand on your partner's yoni and one hand on her chest where her heart is located, and breathe together.

3 Gently and slowly caress her yoni upward, gradually letting two fingers slide between the inner and outer labia on the upward stroke. The fingers should circle around the clitoris, not giving any direct stimulation to it.

4 Pluck at little tufts of her pubic hair with your fingertips. Start gently, checking with your partner frequently to find out how hard she wants you to pull. This sends tiny electrical charges from the pubic mound up through her entire body, which most women find to be very stimulating.

5 Squeeze together the lips of her yoni, with a slow, but firm kneading motion. Pinch gently and rub the outer labia; tugging also feels good in this area of the yoni.

6 Circle your finger between her inner and outer labia in an oval shape, moving from the perineum to above the clitoris.

7 Stroke upward with three fingers; the middle one glides up, slightly inside the yoni opening, and the other two, move on either side. Repeat several times and let her relax into it.

8 Move to pleasure the pearl (clitoris). Start by imagining a clock face around the clitoris. Rub gently and press on each "hour" position around the clock. Go around a few times, varying the speed and pressure to suit your partner.

9 Ask permission to enter her sacred space. Tease at the opening gently with your fingers until she wants to draw your fingers inside. Move one finger in and out, extremely slowly.

10 You can use your fingertips or sides of your fingers to massage the internal four walls of her yoni cave. Alternate this with clitoral stimulation, using your fingers.

11 Ask your partner if she wishes to climax or not. Some women will want to, others won't. There is no right or wrong. Respect her wishes.

12 Finish in stillness. Rest your hands on her yoni and her heart. Tune in with her breathing again. Feel gratitude for your gorgeous partner who welcomed you to her sacred space.

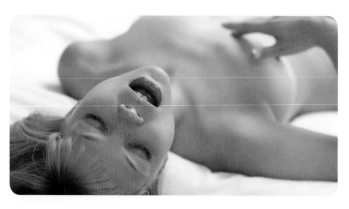

☻ Your cosmic orgasm

Feel free to express yourself fully as you receive a yoni massage. Make sounds and let yourself go. This is sexual healing at its best. Your partner is strong enough to hold the space for you, so ride the waves, then release yourself into a full-body, emotional orgasm. If tears come, let them. If you feel anger or laughter, or any other emotion, let your feelings come out.

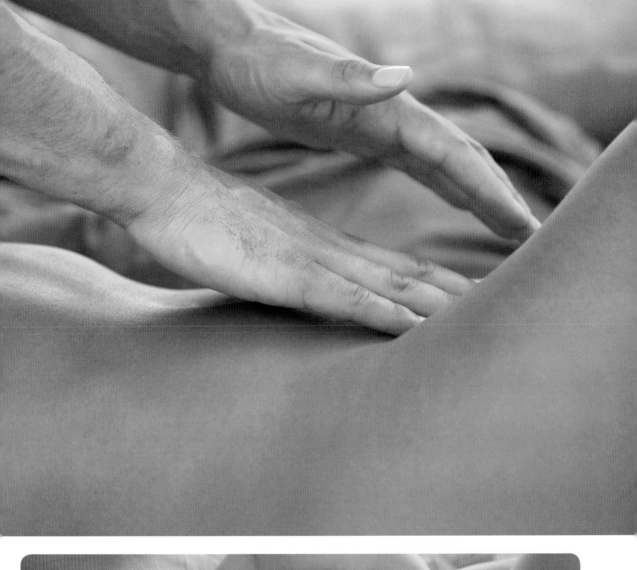
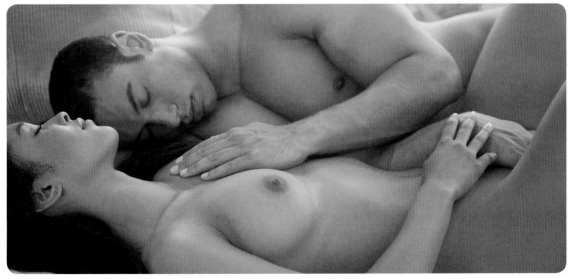

Tantric oral pleasuring

Oral sex is one of the most intimate acts you can engage in with your partner. We all have a deep longing to be intimate with another person. To find this kind of intimacy is possible, but you have to be willing to become emotionally available to your partner.

intimate oral

Pleasuring your partner is a tantric meditation in itself. Oral sex is perfectly designed to bring you both in touch with the moment, encouraging you to live in the present, in harmony with your lover. Oral pleasuring is a very isolated activity; your full attention is given to one point on your partner's body, and you can focus completely on your partner's reactions. Like no other sex act, oral allows you to dwell fully in the moment and on your partner's sensual pleasure.

If you're in any way squeamish about oral sex, this is the perfect opportunity to investigate and drop some of your preconceived notions. Tantra looks upon the human form as the manifestation of the divine, and encourages you to acknowledge and celebrate the beauty in every part, genitals included. Start these meditations with a hot shower together, and feel excitement at the thought of trying something sexy and deeply pleasurable. Jump in and enjoy, remembering that tantra is also known as the "Great Experiment."

vulnerable tantra

During oral sex the giver and receiver are both in a vulnerable position, and it's a chance to develop and instil trust, creating a lasting bond between two lovers. Letting go of your ego and trusting your partner is important in tantra; this loss of ego and control can carry both partners into the still point of unity and pure enlightenment.

The more often you and your partner pleasure each other, the more fully you will know each other, moving together toward ecstasy and divine love. You will actually experience your bodies dissolving in bliss.

๑ Honor your partner

During mutual oral pleasuring, imagine love pouring through your body and into your partner through your touch. As your partner does the same, you create a circle of energy that builds between you. Visualize honoring and worshiping your partner. Remind yourself throughout that your oral pleasuring technique is not all-important: if you perform the act with love, it will shine through.

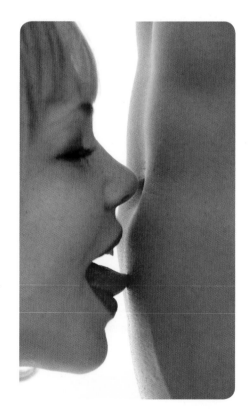

oral sharing

This meditation is an opportunity to express your innermost thoughts and desires. Sharing your truth, uncensored, while engaged in the intimate act of oral pleasuring shows courage and a willingness to take risks, which can be a real turn-on. This can take oral pleasuring to new heights of sensation. You don't need to try and analyze what you're hearing; simply hearing your partner shows empathy.

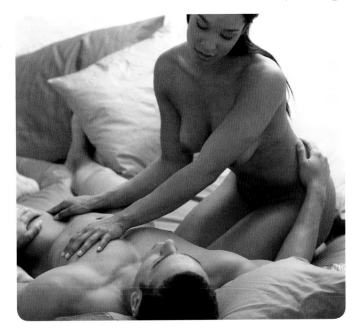

1 Make sure your sacred space is warm. Perform the opening ritual (see page 12).

2 The woman places her hands on her partner's lingam and chest, sending energy to the chakras. Begin to pleasure him orally; there is no need to make anything happen. Remain present and aware by tuning in to your own sensations, and remember to breathe. Relax your throat and mouth as you pleasure.

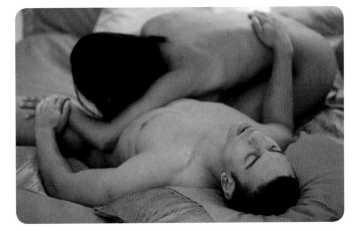

3 During the pleasuring, the man should say whatever comes into his mind. One word might be all; it doesn't have to make sense. The woman does not need to respond; just continue to pleasure him. Receive his words like a gentle wave breaking over you.

4 After five minutes change around, so the woman is receiving the oral pleasuring and sharing her inner experience out loud. Don't discuss what was said, or what happened.

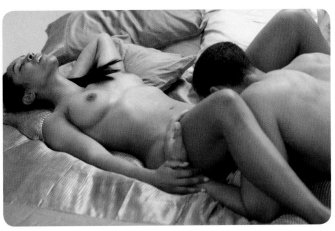

5 If you both desire, move into lovemaking at the end of the pleasuring. Continue to think about the idea of honoring your partner.

6 Perform the closing ritual (see page 12).

worshiping the wand of light

The following meditation is an opportunity to ritualize the pleasuring of your partner's lingam, creating a spiritual experience for both partners. For the man, it is a sublime, nurturing gift. For the woman, imagine that your partner's wand of light is penetrating your body with light energy that caresses your womb and yoni.

1 Sit opposite one another. Chant the sound "Ah" together for five minutes. Open your throat as you tone in unison. See how relaxed you can let your throats become. Laugh together, exaggerating the sounds as your throat relaxes.

2 Hum the universal sound "Om" together for five minutes (see page 98), allowing cosmic energy to fill your being. Feel your body vibrating with vitality and fresh oxygen.

3 Ask your partner to blinfold you, then to lie down and make himself comfortable. Let your tongue investigate the body of your love god. Allow a feeling of respect and awe to envelop you as you touch your partner.

4 When you reach your partner's lingam, perceive it as a wand of light, containing immense healing power and energy. Begin to gently kiss his lingam, and notice how he responds.

5 Run your tongue up and down, and over the head of his lingam. Cradle his testicles gently in one hand.

6 Take your partner's lingam into your mouth with sweet tenderness. For a while, simply enjoy the rising and falling of his energy, and the physical expansion and contraction of his lingam. Tune in to the personality of your partner's lingam; it does have one! Start to move your mouth to pleasure him.

7 The man should remain as still as possible, breathing and enjoying the sensations. The giver should let her mouth receive him and allow her throat to relax. Move your mouth to caress his lingam. Don't rush, stay in each moment. See how expanded and surrendered you can remain throughout.

8 Don't take your Shiva to orgasm; let him surf the waves of pleasure. Let him learn to enjoy every moment.

9 Sit up and take off your blindfold. Rest one hand on his lingam and with the other, stroke small clockwise circles around the top of his head, facilitating an opening in his crown chakra. The man should squeeze his body, then relax and let the sexual energy spread throughout his body.

VITAL SEMEN

In tantra we encourage the man to retain his semen, as a force of life-giving energy. To spill it through ejaculation is considered draining of his energy and male power. Instead, we teach men to try to control their orgasm, keeping the sexual energy generated during self-pleasuring, oral pleasuring, and sexual intercourse inside the body.

At the point of orgasm, a man uses various methods (see above and page 132) to channel his sexual energy throughout his body, to achieve a full-body orgasm. This also means that he can recover more quickly, and resume lovemaking, if desired.

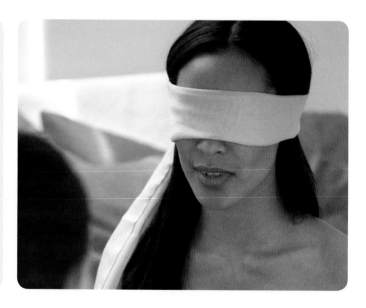

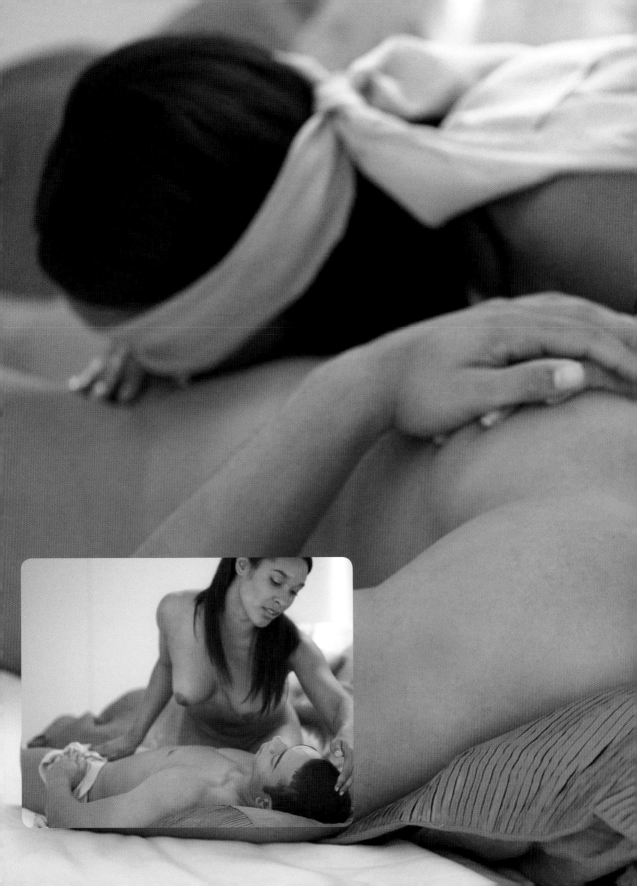

kissing the yoni

Nothing makes a woman feel more adored than having her yoni worshiped by a man who relishes licking, tasting, and feeling her. And any man who indulges in this art with passion knows how the pleasure she experiences transmits directly to his own body. When a woman can allow herself to surrender to sexual pleasure, she experiences a profound sense of liberation, carrying this feeling of freedom into her daily life.

1 Invite your goddess to make herself comfortable, and to open her legs, revealing the entrance to her yoni.

2 Sit for five minutes, and with soft yin vision (see page 108), see her vulva as the heavenly gates to bliss. Kiss her thighs and lower belly slowly and lovingly, feeling desire arise.

3 As you bring your mouth to her sacred place, sense the charge between your tongue and the lips of her yoni.

4 Let your tongue caress between the folds of her outer and inner labia, exploring her folds as if for the first time.

5 Lightly flick your tongue around her pearl (clitoris). Be gentle at first, as some women prefer less direct stimulation until they reach full arousal. Listen to the sounds your partner makes, as they will guide you in the pressure and pace she desires. It will change, moment by moment.

6 Bring your full attention to the tip of your tongue, tuning in to the 3,000 nerve endings that make up the clitoris. Pleasure the pearl with a circular motion of your tongue, increasing the pace as your beloved surfs the waves of ecstasy.

7 Place a hand on your partner's chest near where her heart is; this expands her orgasmic potential and helps her to integrate the sexual energy into her entire body.

8 Just after her climax, turn the pace and pressure right down. Feel the tide receding and ride the waves with her, softening your stroke, all the way to stillness. Rest your head on her belly and breathe together in bliss.

LOTUS NECTAR

In tantra we consider the sexual juices that arise from the yoni (also known as the "living fountain" or "papaya") to be profoundly life-enhancing, containing desirable healing and rejuvenating properties.

When mixed with a man's saliva during oral pleasuring, the combination of these juices becomes a potent elixir. Arouse your beloved and at the same time, savor her yoni's precious secretions, which in tantra we call "lotus nectar". They are considered to be a powerful aphrodisiac, and can enhance your personal sexual enjoyment.

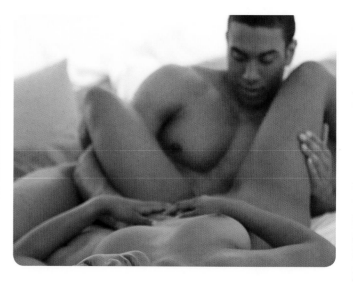

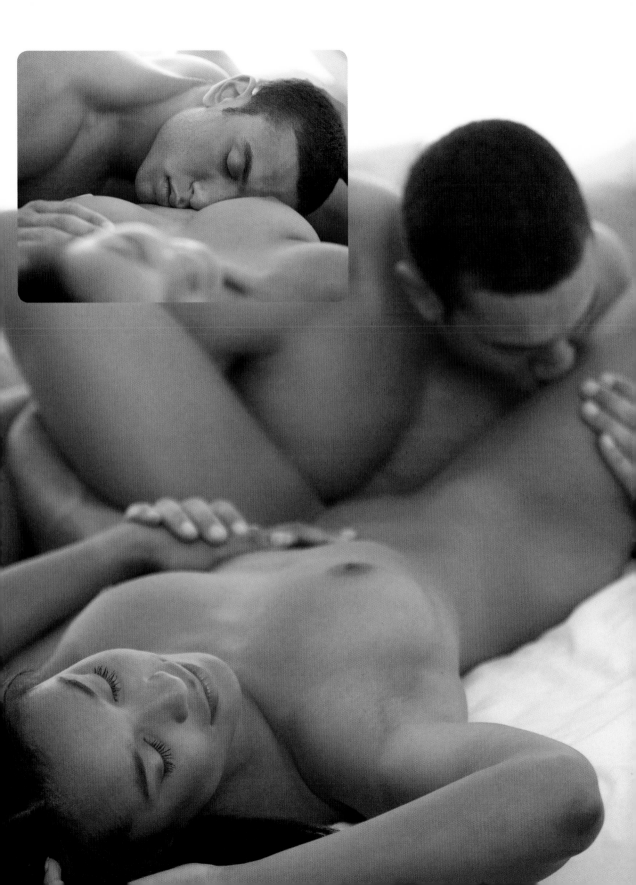

Mutual oral pleasuring

When you pleasure each other's genitals by mouth at the same time, the sexual charge generated becomes a loop between you, creating a circle of rising energy and passion. The sexual energy that grows between you spirals, taking you both toward mutual orgasmic bliss.

enlightened pleasure

Mutual oral pleasuring is one of the fullest representations of the harmony that is possible between the masculine and feminine principles. It can bring a satisfying sense of balance to a couple, with both giving and receiving equally, just as Shiva and Shakti did. The more you and your partner pleasure each other, the more you understand what makes each other aroused and filled with pleasure. Oral pleasuring can make you a master in your partner's physical desires, and is a key part of tantric practice. In time, you may find that oral pleasuring is sexier and even more intimate than sexual intercourse.

☽ Experiencing orgasmic bliss

During tantric oral pleasuring, you can become extremely orgasmic throughout your whole body. Allow the sex energy that's generated through this oral banquet in your genitals to flood your entire body. Let shaking move through you in waves, and surrender to bliss on a cellular level. If genital climax happens to occur, welcome it also, riding the waves of that particular ecstasy.

sideways crow

Featured also in the *Kama Sutra*, this classic position (also known as "69") is fairly easy to get in to, and allows both partners to relax. Once you are in a comfortable position you can both fully relax and immerse yourselves in the tantric experience. Use pillows to raise your heads or buttocks if you need to.

1 Lie on your sides in an inverted position, as shown.

2 Reach through to cradle your partner's buttocks or lower back, to help you stay in position during the meditation.

3 Start by taking turns: the woman can pleasure her partner while he rests his mouth on her yoni, then change so that he pleasures her while she keeps her mouth on his lingam.

4 Move into pleasuring at the same time. Move back and forth between mutual and individual stimulation to heighten the feelings, have time to rest and enjoy the ebb and flow of ecstacy, and to make the pleasuring last as long as possible.

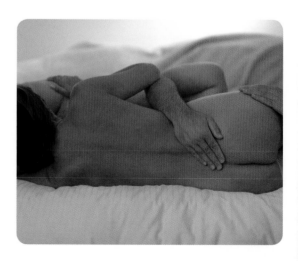

shiva dominant

This is a masculine, sexy variation of oral pleasuring, with the man on top. Take care not to collapse onto your partner as you start to be immersed in the pleasuring. Stay strong throughout, and both rest when you need to.

1 The woman lies down with her head on pillows, and the man kneels above her on all fours, with his knees near her head, and slightly to the side of her body.

2 The man slides his hands underneath his partner's hips to raise her up slightly, and uses his fingers to stimulate her yoni. Use your tongue to pleasure her pearl (clitoris). Use gentle movements at first, building the pressure slowly.

3 The woman then turns her head slightly to find her partner's lingam. Use your hands and mouth to stimulate him. Relax and both savor the mutual pleasuring.

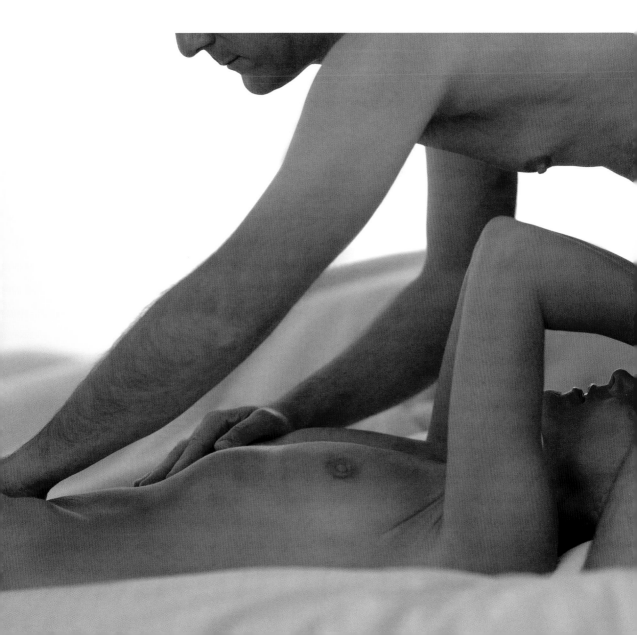

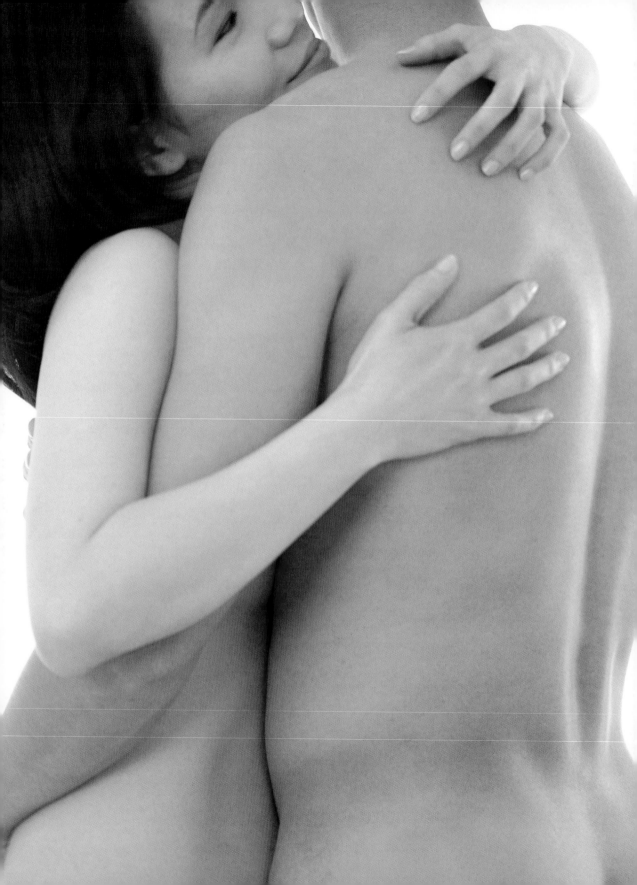

8

ENGAGING THROUGH SEXUAL UNION

The ultimate goal of tantric sex is for both lovers to become one with the divine energy that fills the universe. During your sexual union, you bring together the wisdom and consciousness of Shiva and the love and compassion of Shakti. This potent combination can take you both to nirvana.

The masculine principle

Tantra helps you discover and fulfil the potential of your masculine power. When you are fully comfortable with your masculinity, you can take your sexual enjoyment to a new level, which is a truly sensual turn-on for your partner, too.

unleash your masculinity

Tantric sex is an opportunity to explore and express your masculinity, to become your authentic self, and to take a dominant role as a lover. It is a real turn-on for a woman to experience her lover embracing his strength and assertiveness, but also remaining sensitive and aware of her needs. In tantra, the masculine principle is a potent, sexy combination of strength, tenderness, and power.

True masculine power is sourced from the third chakra (located in the solar plexus) where your energy lines meet. This is where your true self, masculine and strong, yet without ego, finds energy which is manifested throughout your whole being. It is an area where unexpressed feelings and emotions can become stuck and this can affect a man's ability to function at his full capacity, not only in relationships and during sex, but also in the world at large. The meditations opposite and on the next page will help you to unleash your masculine nature.

The more confident a man is in expressing feelings to his partner, the sexier he is. In tantra you are encouraged to express your thoughts, feelings, and desires. If you need time to get comfortable with this, start by imagining yourself as a confident, masculine lover. Visualization can become reality.

remaining present

The desire for penetrative sex can be a driving force in men, and this can impede their creativity in the act of lovemaking. Tantra encourages you to remain present in the moment, giving yourself over to each sensation and movement. You'll find that your moment-to-moment creativity enhances the pleasure of lovemaking for you both, and ultimately enhances your orgasm.

☞ Delaying ejaculation

During lingam massage or sex, your partner can also help you to retain your sexual energy. Here are three methods she can use:

- Grasp the lingam and press your thumb firmly against the point just below the glans. Continue holding until the energy subsides.
- Press firmly into the perineum (the area between the testicles and rosetta). At the same time, place two fingers on the crown chakra and massage in small, continuous circles.
- Rest one hand lightly on the lingam and use two fingers to massage small circles on his heart chakra, between his nipples.

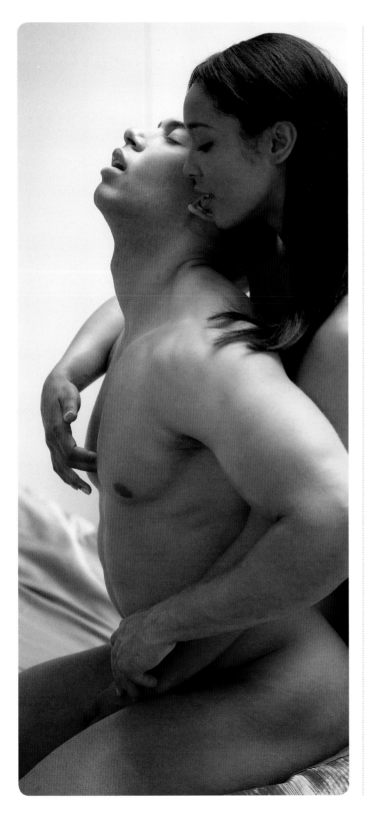

unveiling the god

This meditation is very empowering for a man. It boosts his confidence tremendously, reminding him of his divine nature and encouraging him to celebrate his physical and sexual beauty.

This ritual can also be performed on the woman. You might like to try "Unveiling the Goddess" at another time.

1 Play some sexy, hypnotic, but unobtrusive music. Approach your partner, and slowly remove his clothes, layer by layer, until he stands before you in his magnificent nakedness. As each area of his body is revealed, bring your awareness to each area. Look at it, and let your appreciation of his body build. Move slowly and with thought so he can relax into the meditation.

2 Ask him to sit down and to get comfortable. He can move to lying down if he likes.

3 Let your hands rest on a part of his body and touch and stroke that place with tenderness. Say the words, "This is the chest of the god," or "These are the thighs of the god" as you caress each area of his body.

4 You can let your declarations of worship be in your own words, and add descriptions, as you wish to, for example, "This is the delicious lingam of the god," or "These are the kissable lips of the god." Take your time and cover every inch of his body letting him know how you admire him and how in awe of his beauty and strength you are.

5 When you finish, rest together. You may wish move into lovemaking, where you both enjoy your partner's heightened masculinity.

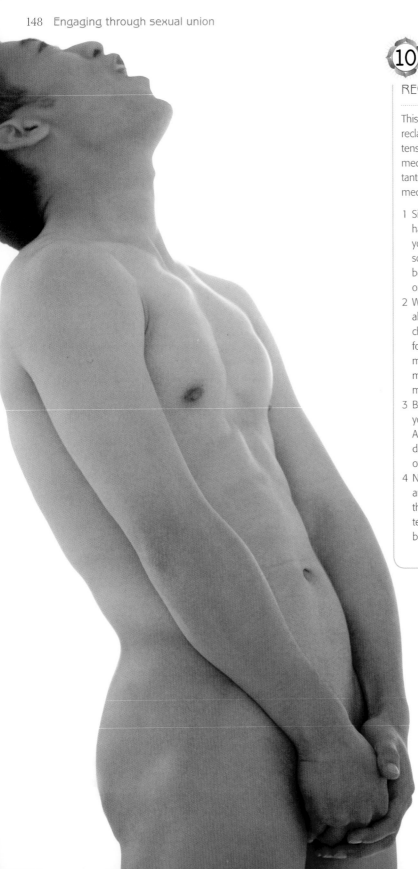

RECLAIM YOUR MANHOOD

This meditation is designed to help you reclaim your masculinity, and to release any tension and repressed feelings. It is a good meditation to try on your own if new to tantra, so you can get more from the meditations with your partner, when ready.

1 Sit or stand comfortably, placing your hands on your genitals. Think back through your life to a situation where you felt someone restricting your energy. It could be a conversation, an argument, a criticism, or something taught to you in school.
2 When you have a picture, shout, "No!" allowing the sound to rise from your base chakra. Then shout, "They're mine!" Sit for a few minutes, feeling the energy move through you. Repeat with any other memory that comes to mind, for up to 10 minutes, until your mind has emptied.
3 Breathe in through your base chakra taking your breath up to the crown of your head. As you breathe out, imagine grace descending over your body like a waterfall of light. Do this for five minutes.
4 Now breathe in through your crown chakra and out through your base chakra, feeling the power flowing in to your lingam and testicles. Your lingam has, quite literally, become a wand of light.

energize your body

You can try this on your own first, and then with your partner. It is designed to increase the positive energy in your base chakra and unleash your masculine power. On your own, imagine that you are making love to the universe. When you try this with your partner, you will both relax in your base chakras, ready for lovemaking.

1 Sit comfortably on your own or opposite your partner. Bring your attention to a point at the root of your lingam. Visualize and sense the energy and power in this area. Feel your pulse rising, and heat moving to that area. Let it pervade your whole being until you resonate with sexual energy.

2 Imagine a circle of energy beginning to loop between your base chakra and your crown.

3 Your partner can sit with her eyes closed, and visualize that she is receiving your masculine energy. She can breathe your energy in through her base chakra, up to her crown, and let cosmic energy rain down over her body.

4 Move into masturbation or lovemaking. Keep your focus on the power emanating from your root chakra and make love from this place of positive, creative energy.

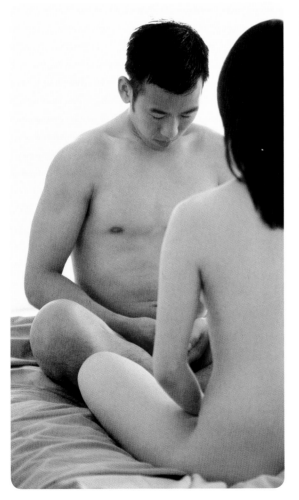

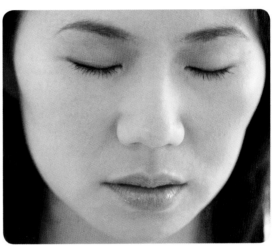

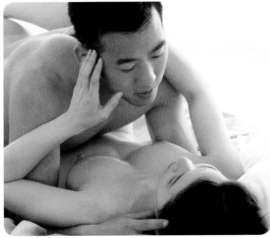

positions that celebrate the masculine principle

Here are a few positions in which a man can assert and express his masculine power during the act of lovemaking. When the man takes a dominant role during sexual union, he accesses his godlike power, and this can act as a potent aphrodisiac for both partners. Always remain aware of your partner's pleasure, by combining sensitivity and tenderness with force and authority to demonstrate your true masculine potential.

penetrate with your eyes

When you feel at the height of your yang male power during sex, it is extremely arousing for your partner if you penetrate her with your eyes, as well as your lingam. Remind yourself to look into her eyes, and show that you are concentrating on her. During more gentle stages, gazing into each other's eyes can also be more conducive to intimacy and spontaneous creativity.

lion position

This position enhances the dynamic of dominance and submission as the man enters the woman's yoni by mounting her from behind. The woman needs to be fully aroused and lubricated for the man to penetrate her in this way.

the plow

The man is on top, and lifts the legs of his partner around his neck. This posture allows for deep penetration, so be sensitive to your goddess and check whether she is comfortable.

man on top

In this position the man can go wild, but he may find that he reaches the point of ejaculation suddenly. If so, move into the Yab Yum position (see page 12) together and breathe into the chakras, until the waves have subsided. Then you can resume.

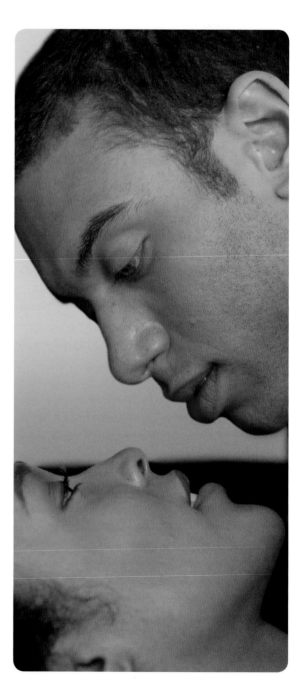

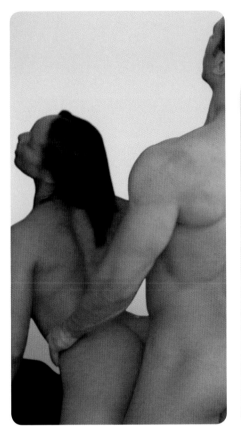

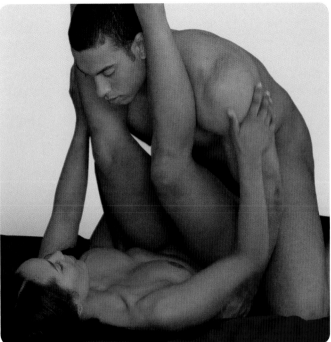

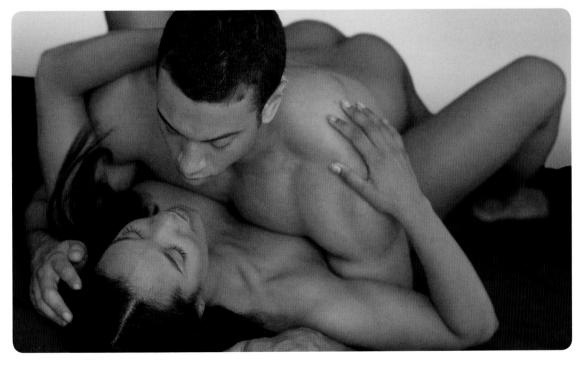

The feminine principle

In tantra every woman is a goddess that embodies the feminine, yin principle of the universe. The more a woman can embrace her true feminine essence during sex, the happier and more fulfilled she will be, and the more she can open to her partner in love.

the feminine mystique

Women carry a sexual mystique and a spiritual wisdom that men are often in awe of. Men dream of a sexually alive woman and find themselves attracted to women who are fully charged with feminine energy. Tantra encourages you to enjoy this potent female sexuality through meditations that give you a safe yet sexy way to explore the full range of feminine sexuality. Meditation will guide you through sexual exploration together, helping you get to know yourself and your partner more fully. When both the feminine and masculine principles meet together in sexual union, the results are sensational.

unleash your feminine power

A woman's sexuality is triggered through love and sensual play. Tantric meditations will help to activate the abundant capacity for orgasm that lies inherent in every woman. The chakras which can best help you to get in touch with your feminine power are the second, fourth, and sixth (see page 20). Massage and attention to these will help to relax and stimulate you.

Be confident in revealing your goddess self during sex. Allow yourself to let go, and to unleash every aspect of your feminine power. Make noise, be fluid and natural in your physicality, allow your emotions to flow freely, and don't be afraid to take charge when the mood comes over you.

Most men respond well to an uninhibited and passionate partner in bed. If your partner is not used to experiencing you in your full capacity as a seductive goddess, he might be surprised at first. Most men, however, will celebrate this as a chance to also step into their own masculine power, and to experiment with a new type of sexual fulfilment.

ꕥ Love your goddess

Sex is a great way to express your love and passion for your partner, but it is not the only way. Tantra encourages you to express your love in both sexual and non-sexual ways, to allow your partner to flourish.

- Listen to your partner, rather than try to fix everything. One of the qualities of the feminine goddess is being emotionally expressive, so show your love for your partner by listening to her. The tantric approach is to "become like a rock that the sea breaks against." This simple act of unconditional acceptance will transform your relationship in every way.
- Show physical affection every day, not just when you want sex. Your partner needs to be reminded on a regular basis how much she's desired, and how adored she is. Stroke her, kiss her, hold her, and share your feelings with her, and you'll find that your intimacy levels soar.
- Make love with full consciousness. Look at her body, feel her body, and make every touch express your love and desire.

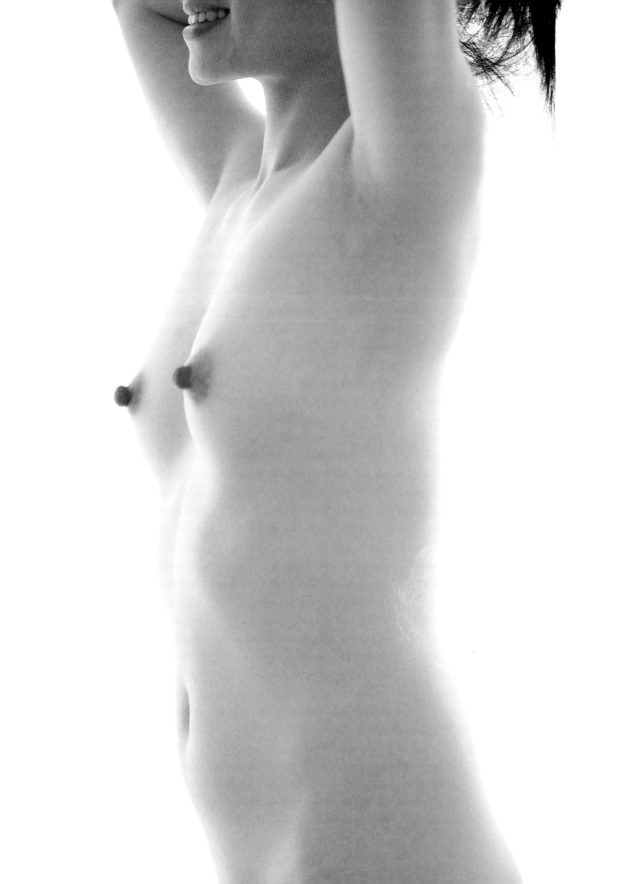

greeting the goddess

This meditation invites you to remember when you discovered your partner for the first time. You see each other through fresh eyes, enjoying each other's bodies anew. The man uses his senses to get to know his partner. This allows the woman to feel and express her femininity, and the man to be overwhelmed by her spirit.

1 The man undresses first, and the woman blindfolds him. She then undresses completely.

2 Stand facing each other. The woman asks the man to step forward. He takes three slow, small steps forward. Stand close, but not touching. The man senses the energy of his partner. After a few minutes he takes three steps back.

3 The woman asks him to step forward again. This time he smells her gently, starting at the neck, and moving to wherever he wants to explore. He could smell her hair, her skin, and between her thighs, if he likes. He steps back.

4 At the next approach, use your sense of touch to greet your goddess. Use slow, reverential touch, unhurried and curious, and explore every curve of her body as if for the first time. Stroke her hair, and feel her face gently.

5 On the next greeting, embrace, and feel your hearts connect as your bodies meet. Then step back again.

6 The woman puts on some erotic dance music and invites the man forward. Ask the man to remove his blindfold. Dance naturally so your partner can watch, revealing your true nature (there is no need to perform).

7 Move into lovemaking, retaining the sense of awe and wonder that arose in the meditation. Let the female sexual energy move you both. Allow the woman to be free, gentle, passionate, and explosive, and don't control her. When you kiss your goddess, experience it as if for the first time. Breathe deeply while you allow her desire to cascade over you in waves. During penetration, allow yourself to disappear as if into a vast chasm, as if making love to the universe.

8 At moments, whenever it feels right, come into stillness and let your eyes wander over the body of your goddess, enjoying her natural beauty and purity of spirit.

9 Allow orgasm to happen, or just rest together, enjoying your new awareness of each other.

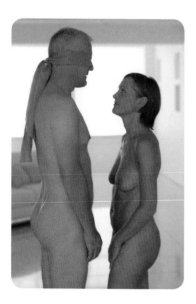
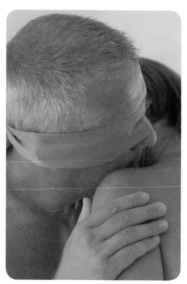
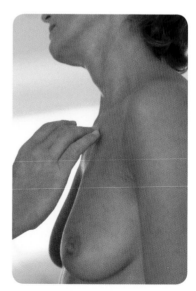

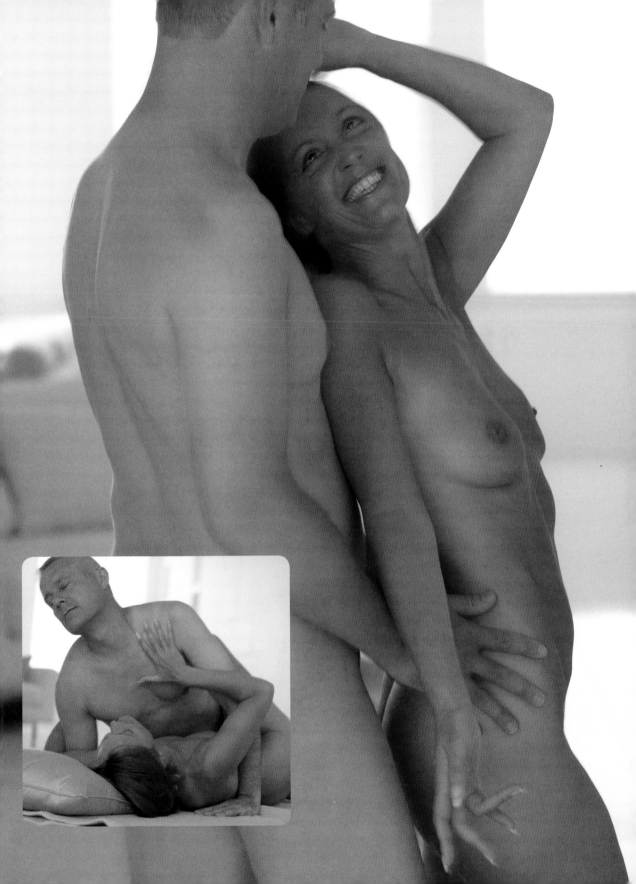

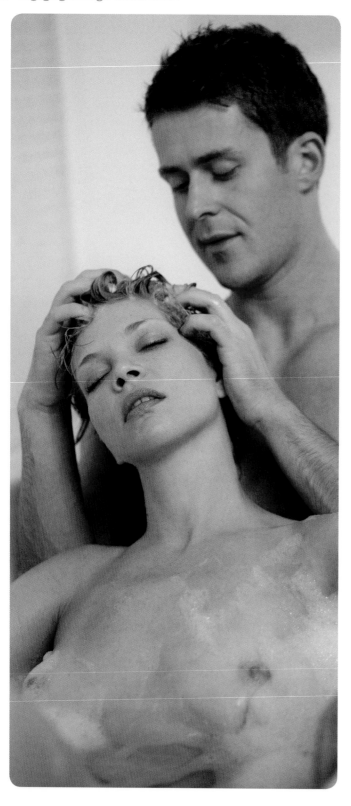

ravishing the goddess

This is an opportunity to really ravish your partner; to make love to her so that every part of her is truly satisfied. If you plan to do this at least once a month, you will reap the benefits a thousandfold. Ravishing your partner doesn't have to be choreographed every time; the magic can happen spontaneously, and each time, your relationship moves to a deeper level of intimacy. Before you start, share a fantastic meal together, and prepare your bedroom with flowers and candles, to make your partner feel divine.

1 Bathe your partner lovingly and wash her hair, massaging her head and rinsing the shampoo away gently. Let her soak in the bath while you sit, relaxed, enjoying her company and beauty. Let her talk, and listen without trying to fix her or offer solutions.

2 Dry your partner and give her a sensuous massage using massage oil, including a yoni massage (see page 134). There is no need to bring her to orgasm at this point.

3 Dance for each other. Enjoy gazing at your partner's body, and see the beauty and divine spirit in each other.

4 Move into lovemaking. Be the masculine yang energy, and give yourself fully to lovemaking. Allow her to expand into her full yin essence. Satiate your beloved with your desire. Let her know with every touch and every kiss that she means more to you than any other woman in the world.

5 After lovemaking comes to a natural end, although preferably not in ejaculation, lie together in bliss. Hold your partner with love.

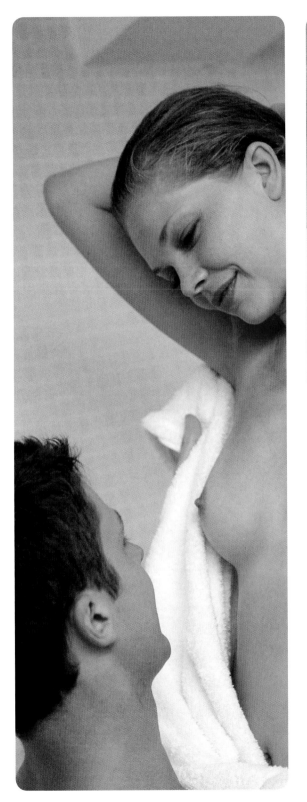

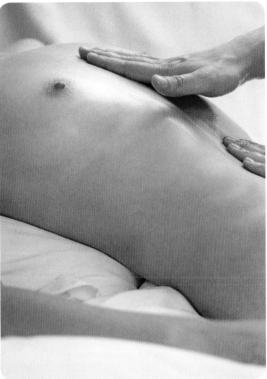

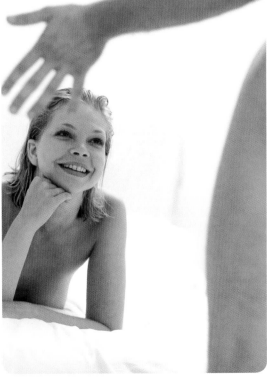

Sexual harmony

When the masculine and feminine forces fully meet during sex, the result are electric. Your sexual and emotional desires will be satisfied in new ways, your senses will feel fully alive, and you will experience an intoxicating sense of passion and connection.

tantric gods and goddesses

In tantric sex, the female embodies every woman in the universe. The man demonstrates his love and trust through spontaneous acts of devotional worship. As a result, the woman opens like a lotus flower, radiating serenity, beauty, and bliss. In response, the man surrenders, allowing ego to die as he drowns in the fullness of his partner's feminine power.

The male partner represents every man in the world, and appears to his beloved as an omnipotent god. The woman submits to his passion, desire, and energy. Shakti opens to her beloved without resistance, discovering her true strength while letting go. The most precious and sensual times you spend together are ones in which you feel free to fully abandon to your divine feminine and masculine selves.

Embracing passion and surrender

If you would like more passion in your love life, think and act passionately, and you'll find yourself creating more of it than you dreamed possible. If you feel that you would benefit from surrendering more in your life, carve out time and space for your body to let go. Create your own reality and paint the canvas of your life. Bring this approach to your sex life, and you will find the impact astounding.

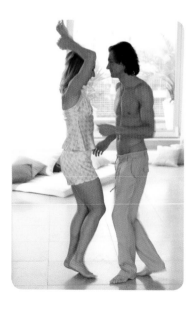
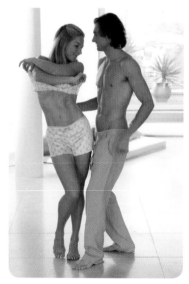
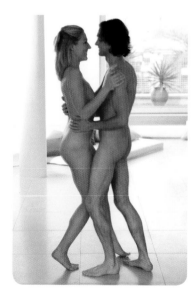

shiva shakti dance

This meditation combines dancing and sex, bringing the energy generated from spontaneous, wild dancing straight into lovemaking. It also helps to balance the masculine and feminine polarities, bringing a sense of deep fulfilment to both the man and the woman. Be total in this meditation and experience the intense and profound merging that can occur when both the masculine and feminine desires are satisfied.

1 Perform the opening ritual (see page 12).

2 Play wild and stimulating dance music and as you dance with each other, remove your clothing until you are completely naked. Watch your partner as you each undress.

3 Allow the sexual energy to rise while you dance. Gyrate your hips, and focus your attention on your genitals, and wake them up with rhythmic movements. Stare into each other's eyes, feeling a yearning for sexual union rising in your body. Dance for five minutes, watching each other.

4 Come together in sexual union, giving yourselves over to animalistic desire. Be total, abandoning yourselves to lust, but don't make genital release the goal. After 10 minutes of making love, allow the pace and intensity to tail off.

5 Come into stillness and as the man's erection diminishes, pull apart and stand up, facing each other again.

6 Play some soft, rhythmic music and dance opposite one another, looking tenderly into the eyes of your beloved. After five minutes of dancing, lay down together in an embrace.

7 Do circular breathing together. The man breathes out of his base chakra, the woman receiving the breath in through her base chakra. The woman breathes out of her heart chakra, and the man receives in through his heart chakra. After five minutes, change the direction of your breathing.

8 Fall into easy breathing, sinking into a deep stillness together, feeling universal light energy pour down through your crown chakras, illuminating your bodies. Rest together.

9 Repeat the meditation as many times as you like. One sequence can be enough to generate a potent harmonization, or you can just go on, getting higher in each yang phase of passion and lovemaking, and finding deeper bliss in the stillness of each yin phase of rest.

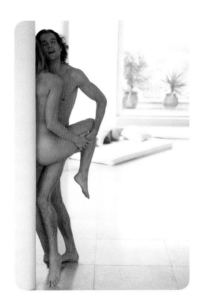

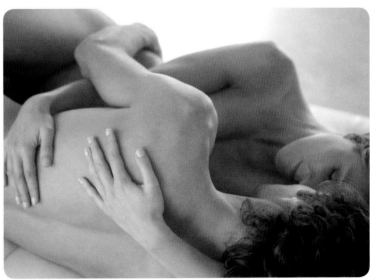

royal liberation meditation

This meditation was designed to help royalty achieve spiritual fulfillment while living a life of worldly activity. Use it to release yourself from daily responsibilities and pressures, and give space to your sexiest desires. This meditation can take all evening, or even all night. The person who is king or queen must ask for all their desires, and feel truly satisfied by the end of the meditation. The next time you perform this exercise, change roles.

1 Perform the opening ritual (see page 12). Decide who will be king or queen. Here, the man is king for the night.

2 The man sits with his eyes closed. The woman kneels at his feet, with a scarf covering her head.

3 Entering a meditative state, the man allows the characteristics of a king to permeate his being, and the woman the qualities of a consort or slave. The woman lets go of personal will, as if she were born to serve her beloved master, and fulfil his every wish.

4 The man imagines that his central channel, which runs from the base chakra to the crown chakra (see page 20) is filling with light, allowing him to attain spiritual awakening.

5 When the man removes her scarf they are fully in role. The king lets a desire arise in his mind. He speaks it out loud while looking into the eyes of his consort. He says, "I want..."

You can ask for the simplest of desires but you must demand them as if it is your birthright. Be creative and ask for things you've never asked for before. Perhaps you would like to feel your hair stroked softly, to hear compliments about your lingam, to be tied to a chair and blindfolded, or to have your consort wear sexy lingerie and dance for you. Let your imagination go wild. Don't censor yourself.

6 Exhaust your desires. If you need to continue all night, that's fine. It's your night. After you have asked for everything you desire and feel utterly satiated, say, "I am complete."

7 Perform the closing ceremony (see page 12), upon which the consort and the king return to their former selves.

8 If you have a garden the man could lie alone under the night sky, meditating on desire, for as long as he is comfortable, basking in his renewed sense of self and in the profound pleasure of being satisfied by his lover.

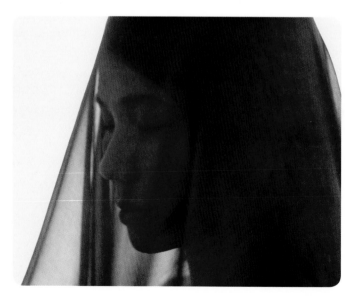

☙ Reflection on desire

Our desires reflect our innermost wants and needs. In our everyday lives, it is rarely appropriate to express our desires in the moment they occur, and we often tend to suppress these feelings. By doing so, however, you may actually be doing yourself a disservice. Through learning to override your emotions, it is possible to become alienated from what you really want or need in order to feel satisfied. Instead of denying your desires as they come to you, make a mental note of them. Later, examine these thoughts with your partner and compare notes on desire. The act of sharing will give you both insight and will make it easier to act on some of these desires together.

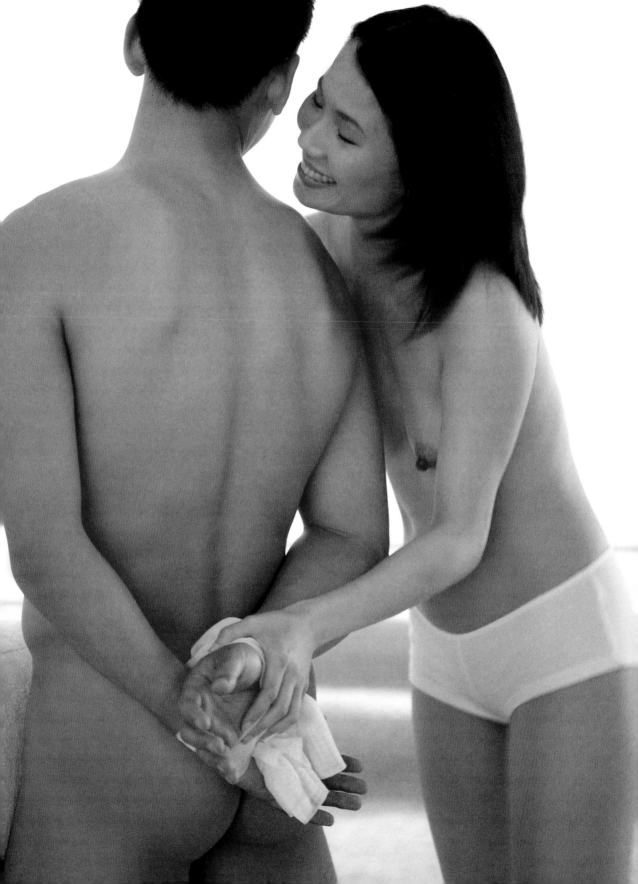

Cosmic orgasm

In tantric sex, orgasm is more than a fleeting physical release. A tantric orgasm brings spontaneous, ecstatic waves of energy that fill your entire body. You may feel a gentle undulation, a thunderbolt of lightning, or earthquake tremors—all intensely pleasurable.

tantric orgasm

Orgasmic energy is the greatest healing force available to us as human beings, and the tantric approach to sex gives you the ability to access it in each and every moment during sex. The universe is in a state of constant orgasm–all you have to do is open up and tap into the ever-flowing source.

Both men and women are capable of achieving a full-body, cosmic orgasm. Often we cheat ourselves for a quick fix, a quick orgasm and ejaculation, but it is your birthright to taste the nectar of true sexual fulfillment. As you re-frame your ideas of how sex should look and feel, you can experience orgasm as a gateway to transcendence, and ultimately as a source of profound healing and refreshment.

During tantric meditation, allow yourselves to follow the flow of energy and emotion that occurs naturally between your bodies without trying to force an outcome. The tantric orgasm happens without effort, technique, or agenda. You are both awake and conscious, yet are in a surrendered state, moving into a state of oneness, where your bodies expand effortlessly to experience completely intimate pleasure.

cosmic orgasm for men

Most men associate orgasm with ejaculation, but compared to the kind of spectacular, full-body orgasm possible during tantric sex, ejaculation is a minor physical function. Through practice, a man can learn to channel his orgasmic energy to fill his entire body. He can surf the waves of orgasmic bliss for hours without ejaculating. He can learn to climax like a woman, drawing his sex energy upward through his central channel, sending it out of his crown chakra like an orgasmic, cosmic geyser.

THE BIG BANG THEORY

One interpretation of the Big Bang theory is that the world started as a giant orgasm that gave birth to the world. Perhaps the world continues to exist as one, long, cosmic orgasm, and we can try to tap into that energy. During our experience of orgasm, we connect with the cosmic energy of the world, and our energy spirals outward to join with it. Simultaneously, it spirals to merge with us, giving our physical union a tangible power.

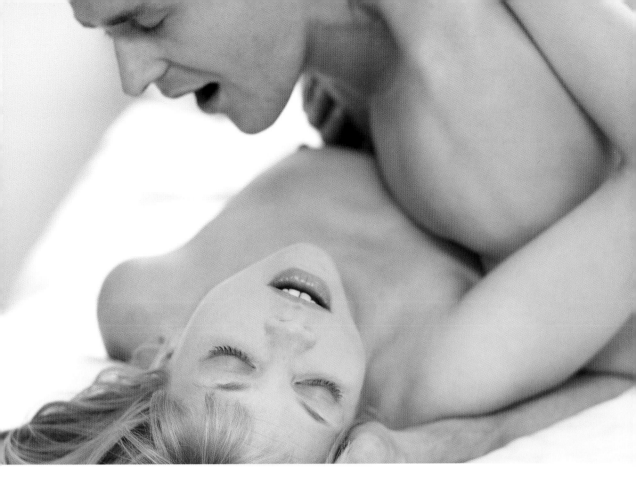

cosmic orgasm for women

It is important for both partners to understand that penetration alone will not make a woman orgasm. Most women need stimulation of the clitoris in order to orgasm, so this should always be part of your sexual union. To intensify orgasm, you can also stimulate vaginal areas like the G-spot, and erogenous zones such as nipples, breasts, neck, and wherever else appeals to your partner. Nerves located in the nipples have a direct link to the clitoris, so this is an especially good place to touch.

During the build-up to orgasm both the interior and exterior of the yoni become engorged and enlarged. The yoni produces secretions and the woman can experience a kind of internal ache, which is a physical longing for penetration. Breathing rate, heart rate, and blood pressure increase, and nipples become erect. If the woman is relaxed and flowing with her energy and emotions, and can let go of control, she will be able to dive into the vast ocean of orgasm, surfing waves of ecstatic bliss.

WHAT DOES ORGASM FEEL LIKE?

A group of tantricas were asked to describe their own orgasm. These evocative descriptions are very similar to those used by people attempting to convey what happens to them in a state of enlightenment. When you combine sex and meditation, you can also experience these amazing feelings.

- Release
- Stream of energy
- Heart explosion
- Bliss
- White water rapids
- Cascade
- Beyond control
- Prisms of light
- Kaleidoscope of shooting stars
- Expanded vision
- Universal love

what women want

Women's sexual energy naturally rises and falls in waves. Unlike the male sex drive, female sexual rhythm is more "go with the flow" than goal-orientated. It is important for partners to note these differences and try to meet each other's needs, both physically and spiritually. When a man chooses to delay orgasm and control ejaculation, he is showing that the focus of his lovemaking is no longer just about the end result. He is there for pleasure, of course, but also to bring mutual sexual and emotional fulfilment to both himself and his partner.

the addiction of ejaculation

Men often become addicted to ejaculation early on in life, because of the quick, intense burst of pleasure that it brings. One common reason for men's compulsion to ejaculate is because it is the only emotional release mechanism they know. When a man is stressed or anxious, ejaculating can bring momentary relief, but not ultimate fulfillment. A man who works toward accessing pleasure on both an emotional and spiritual level will gain full control over his sexual energy. Practicing tantric meditations will help bring the goal of sex away from ejaculation, and toward more rewarding emotional and sexual release. Many men find that once they break this habit they achieve awe-inspiring cosmic orgasms.

☙ Staying connected after sex

After ejaculation, there is sometimes a desire in the man to withdraw, becoming separate from his partner. This is natural in men and they are not to be criticized for it. One of the positive consequences of the man refraining from ejaculating is that he will experience less desire to move away or fall asleep after sex. This means that you can stay emotionally and spiritually connected for some time, cherishing your emotional connection and resting peacefully together in post-orgasmic bliss.

controlling your ejaculation

During sex if you feel close to ejaculation, try one or more of these methods to retain semen. It can take time to master these methods, but let your body get used to the new ways of moving sexual energy, at your own pace. Your partner can help with some of the techniques.

1 Relax and take your focus away from your genitals. Visualize your orgasmic energy moving up through your body. As you breathe in, visualize your sexual energy drawing upward, flowing toward your heart. As you breathe out, release it from your heart chakra, into your partner's heart.

2 Move into the Yab Yum position (see page 12), keeping your lingam inside your partner. Breathe and sway together, keeping your close connection, but allowing the dip in energy to relax your body and extend your arousal.

3 Squeeze your pubococcygeal muscles tight (these are the muscles that you use if you want to stop the flow of urine) and take a deep, sharp intake of breath.

4 Press on the point just below your glans and hold it until the urge to ejaculate subsides. Press firmly into the indentation on the perineum.

5 Gently massage your testicles, then stroke down your thighs and up your belly toward your heart.

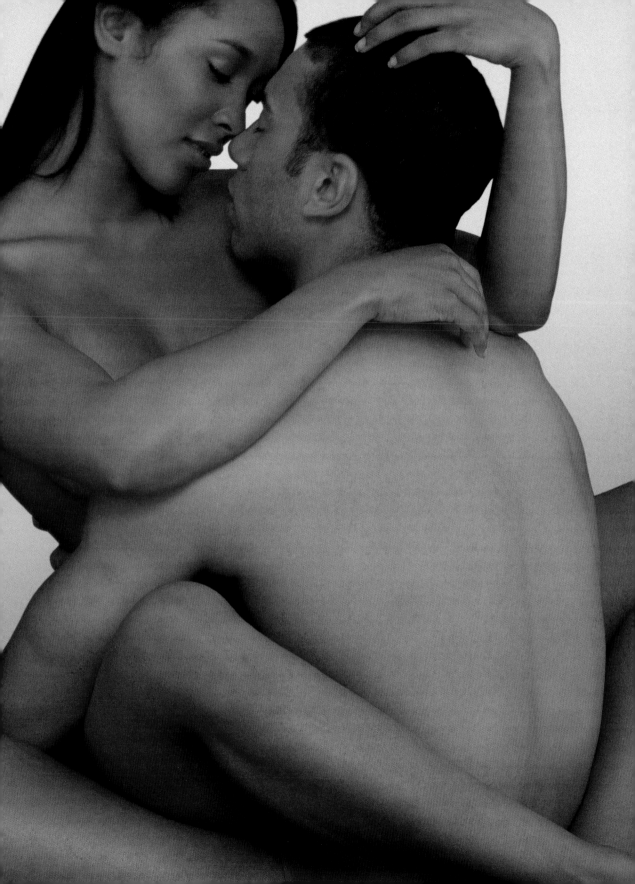

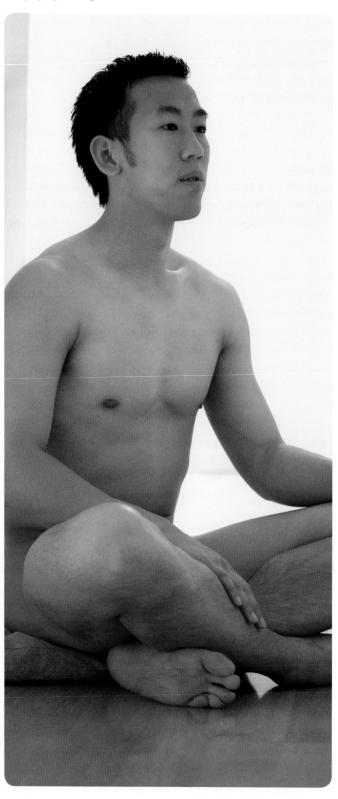

toning the love muscles

To experience more powerful orgasms and to increase your sexual desire and stamina, try these exercises to strengthen your pelvic floor muscles. Both men and women can benefit from them. If you practice this simple method daily, you are guaranteed to intensify your orgasms.

It may take a while to distinguish between the two sets of muscles, but as they gain strength, you will find it easier. Never do more than 60 contractions, otherwise the pelvic floor area can become too rigid.

1 Sit or stand comfortably. As you breathe in, squeeze your anus, keeping the rest of your genital area relaxed. Breathe out and relax. Repeat 10 times.

2 Breathe in deeply and hold your breath. Squeeze your genitals, making sure that the muscles in your anus are relaxed. Breathe out and relax. Repeat five times.

☺ Make some noise

Sound is one way of increasing the intensity of your orgasm. Allow yourself to make spontaneous sounds, and your whole being, body and soul, can become orgasmic. You may laugh, cry, or even scream from the depths of ecstasy. Allow yourself to let go and encourage your partner to do the same.

learn from your partner

In this arousing meditation you each allow the other to watch you self-pleasuring. This gives you the opportunity to demonstrate what turns you on, and show how you like to reach orgasm. Take turns to show and watch. The mutual understanding that arises from this ritual will greatly enhance your lovemaking.

1 Get comfortable together in your sacred space.

2 While one partner self-pleasures, the other should watch using receptive yin vision (see page 108). Allow your gaze to soften, and observe without scrutiny or comment. It is better not to talk during this ritual, so as not to lose the energy.

3 After reaching orgasm, allow your partner to hold you, silently sharing the intimate space together.

4 Exchange roles. Afterward, share what you learned from observing each other. Verbalizing what you've seen takes a special kind of vulnerability, but can also be very erotic.

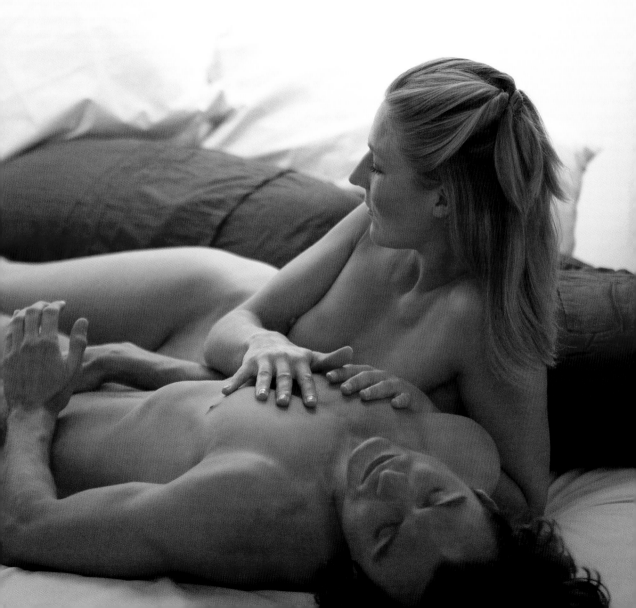

peaks and valleys

This lovemaking meditation takes you on an incredible journey through the peaks and valleys of sexual passion and energy, building toward cosmic orgasm together. During the valley parts of the meditation, allow yourselves to rest completely, even sleeping if you want. During the peak parts, rise together in passion and desire.

1 Perform the opening ceremony (see page 12).

2 Begin to make love, allowing the sexual energy to grow naturally and easily. The man should be attentive and loving toward his partner, allowing her arousal to awaken without effort. Make love for about 20 minutes, and allow yourself to be active and creative. Fuel the fire with deep breathing and lots of eye contact. If the man feels the desire to ejaculate, use the methods on page 164 to move beyond ejaculation.

3 At this time, you may feel a natural dipping of sexual energy and decrease of passion. Allow yourselves to sink into an inactive state together. Relax and surrender into the yin space, remaining there for another 20 minutes without moving. To retain your connection, the man's lingam should stay inside the woman's yoni, and become soft.

4 Feel the sexual energy rising again. It should not be forced, but should come from a place deep inside you. Make love, moving into an even higher peak of ecstasy. Be free and wild if you wish; let universal energy move you.

5 After 20 minutes, relax together again. Again after 20 minutes, let the energy rise naturally, making love passionately, without holding back any desires.

6 Allow yourselves to become one in ecstasy. Let go and let orgasm take over your bodies, feeling every cell alive and vibrating. If the man feels like ejaculating, he can choose to release in this way, or not.

7 Rest together in silence. After 20 minutes, perform the closing ceremony (see page 12).

☯ Arousing your partner

Women can take at least 20 minutes to reach a state of arousal and readiness for penetration. When you allow your Shakti as much time as she needs to open sexually, she will reach higher states of ecstasy during intercourse.

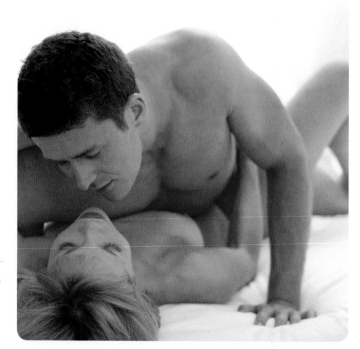

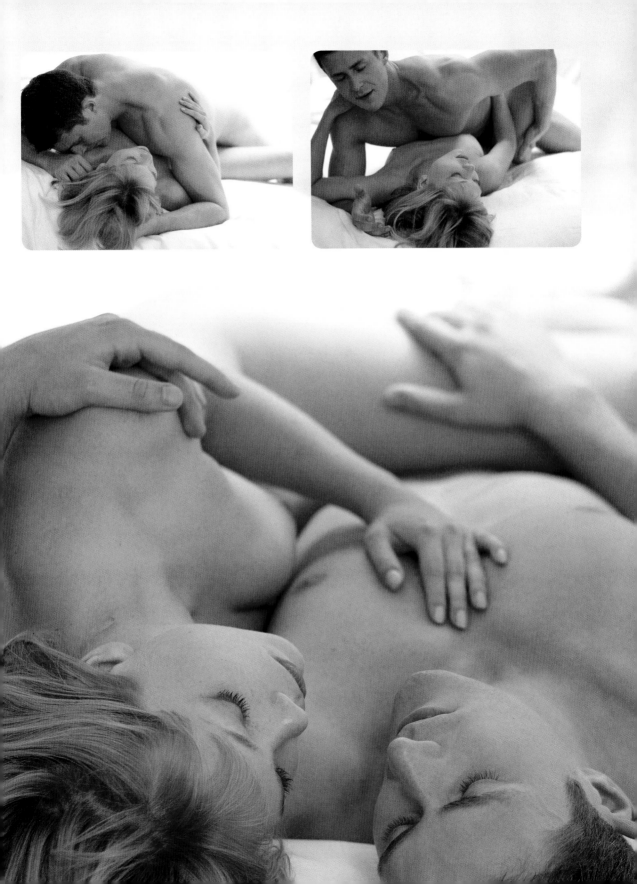

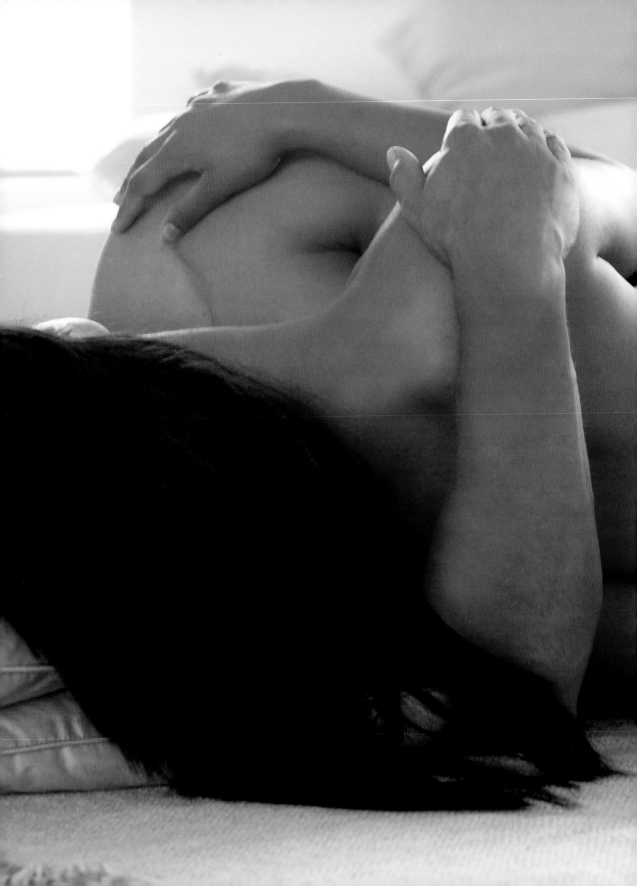

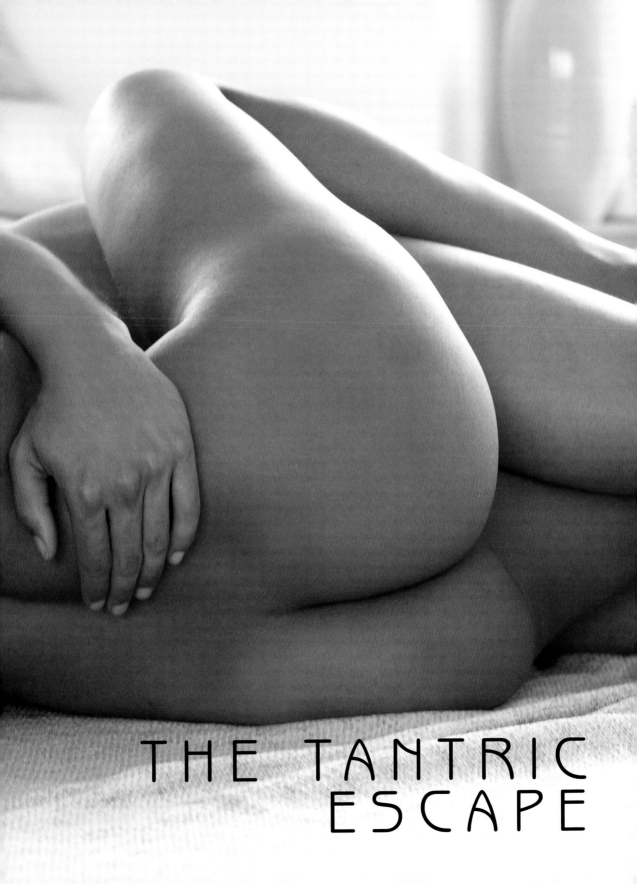

THE TANTRIC
ESCAPE

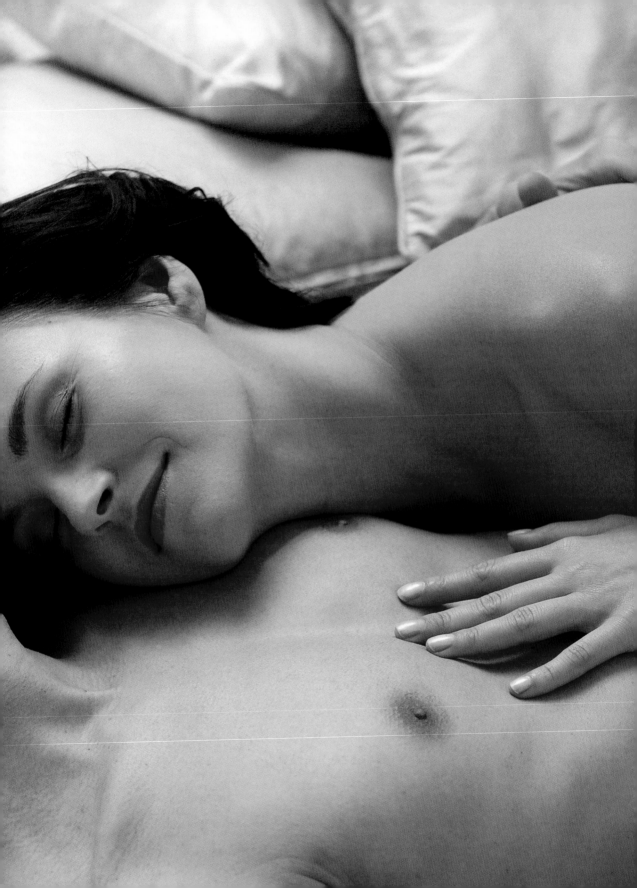

9

THE TANTRIC RETREAT

One of the best things you can do for your relationship is to plan time away together for intimacy, love, and sex. Take this time to rediscover your partner and use it as an opportunity to fully experience new tantric meditations together. In this environment, lovemaking can happen without effort, unfolding in a relaxed, sensual, and satisfying way.

Planning your retreat

Your sexy tantric weekend away can be as inventive as you like. Plan every moment, or be spontaneous—just make it a time of indulgence, intimacy, and exploration. You may want to revisit some of your favorite meditations from this book, or try something for the first time.

where to go

It doesn't really matter where you end up; the tantric energy you are going to create together will make any location special. One important factor is that the venue should be conducive to making lots of noise, such as a private cottage in the country. You want to feel relaxed and uninhibited. Your venue doesn't have to be luxurious, but it does have to be warm and comfortable. Spa facilities and a garden are an added bonus, and somewhere that can provide room service or an in-room kitchen will make it easy to indulge in sensually private meals.

Osho centers are located around the world and can provide wonderful settings for tantric indulgence. They are used to visitors expressing themselves in an uninhibited way, so you will not feel self-conscious. Some centers will even prepare you an aphrodisiac dinner for an erotic blindfold meal.

before you go

Sit down together and talk about what you'd both like to get out of your weekend away. Share your ideas without censoring,, and fire each other up with new desires and longings.

Remember to listen: if you want to stay in and take a long bath, and he wants to get outside for a long walk, you will need to be flexible. You don't have to fit everything in to one weekend; allow time for spontaneity. The higher the expectations, the greater the pressure to perform, so make sure you don't create an overly ambitious agenda.

If it seems difficult to plan time away, remember that when you return from a tantric break, refueled with energy, positivity, and love, you will carry the benefits into every area of your life.

PACKING YOUR BAGS

You should bring with you any items you find especially sensual: clothing in luxurious fabrics, sexy music, massage oil, feathers, an erotic movie or two. Use this checklist as a basis, then add to it with your own favorites:

- music and small stereo
- lubricant and massage oil
- incense and aromatherapy oils
- blanket or sheet to lie on during massage
- erotic literature and movies that you will both enjoy
- blindfolds or silk scarves
- feathers

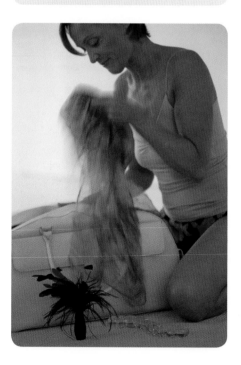

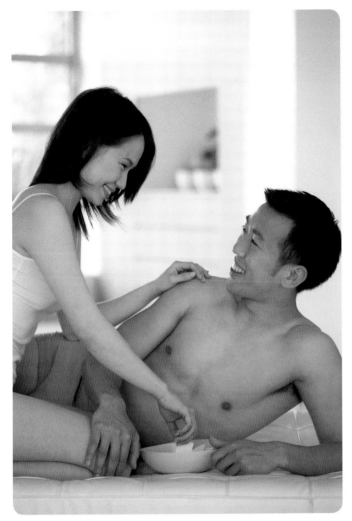
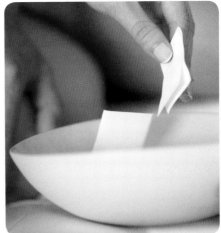
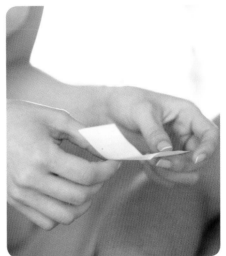

choose your activities

This meditation is a nice way to agree what to do on your weekend. It is especially useful if time is limited. Write down anything you like to do with your partner, from oral sex to sharing a leisurely breakfast. Combining both of your thoughts should give you a wide range of activities. Anything that is mentioned twice is a definite yes.

1 Tear up some paper into small pieces (about 20 should do).

2 Sit down opposite each other and fill each piece of paper with one activity you'd like to indulge in on your tantric break. Be as creative as you like.

3 Place the pieces into a large bowl centered between you.

4 Take it in turns to take an option out of the bowl and read it out loud to your partner. Keep an open mind as you consider each option.

5 If there are any surprises, talk them over together. Decide together if you would like to try them, or agree to see how you feel about them on your retreat.

Day one

Enjoy the sense of anticipation that you both feel as you leave on your retreat. Don't plan too much for this evening. Allow yourselves to relax, get acquainted with your new surroundings, and revel in the chance to spend extended time alone together.

setting the scene

This is the afternoon or evening that you arrive at your destination. When you have both eaten and had a glass of wine, set the tone for the weekend by giving each other a sexy massage. This one is designed to relax you both, shed the tensions of the week, and get your chakras spinning.

If you are both full of energy and excitement, move into lovemaking afterward. If you both need to sleep, the power that has been generated through the massage will help to energize and revive you throughout the night, and prepare you to fully engage in the next day's plans.

☉ Switch off

Make a promise to each other to turn off your cell phones so that your time together is uninterrupted. You may agree to allocate one hour each day to check for messages, if you feel you need to. Keep the time as short as possible – it is healthy to discover how everyone manages without you.

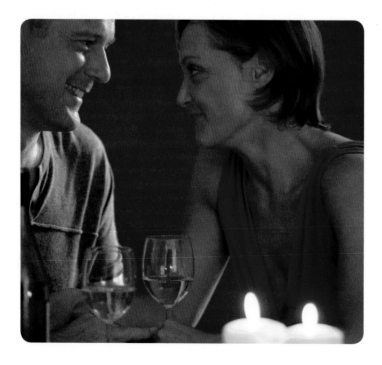

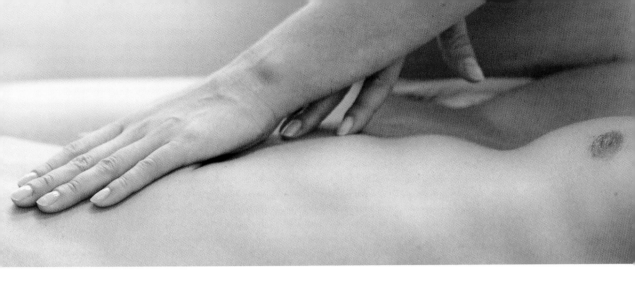

positive pole massage

This sexy massage brings you into alignment with your partner and enhances the magnetism between you by awakening your three "positive" poles. After you finish, you will both be in a place of heightened sensitivity, with your hearts fully open. You can follow this with lovemaking, or simply rest together.

1 Ask your partner to lie on his front. Massage his back, concentrating on his first positive pole, the sacrum (his lower back) and guiding that energy up the spine. Massage his head and then the back of the legs and feet.

2 Ask your partner to turn over. Massage his belly with clockwise movements around his navel. Rest your hands for a few moments on his solar plexus (the second positive pole) and breathe in time with your partner. This will deepen your connection, aligning your spirits and your bodies.

3 Stroke upwards, over his chest and shoulders and down his arms and hands. This takes the energy from the third chakra into the whole body. Massage his arms and hands.

4 Massage his neck and throat gently. Rest one hand on his throat (the third positive pole) and the other on the back of the neck. Massage his head, including his face and scalp.

5 Massage around his groin area and focus on the sensitive perineum point between his testicles and anus. Next, massage his lingam and testicles, and cradle them gently in your hands (see page 132).

6 To finish the massage, stroke down his legs and then up his body, over his chest and down the arms. Rest while your partner relaxes completely.

7 Change places so the woman is lying on her front. Follow the same massage techniques, until you reach her chest. A woman's first positive pole is found in her lower belly, so massage gently in circles to activate.

8 The second positive pole is found near the heart. Massage her chest gently in upward sweeping strokes, between the breasts and toward her throat. Rest your hand on her heart. With the other hand, gently massage between her eyebrows to activate her third positive pole. Then, massage her breasts. Visualize honoring her as a goddess; you are not trying to arouse her (see page 156).

9 Massage softly around her yoni and pubic hair (see page 134), with great adoration and respect. Stroke down her legs, then up and over her chest to her arms and hands to take the energy through her entire body.

10 Rest while your partner relaxes completely.

Day two

Today is your opportunity to devote time to each other. Live in the moment, enjoying each other's company, and indulging in whatever makes you both feel relaxed and uninhibited. You may want to start the day with sex, or build anticipation for the evening.

a day of indulgence

This day should be about enjoying the presence of your partner in every way. Indulge in the opportunity to spend uninterrupted time in each other's company. No matter how long your relationship, you have chosen each other for a reason, and you may want to begin the day reflecting on what you appreciate about your partner and sharing these thoughts with him or her.

Spend the day engaged in relaxing and renewing activities that you both enjoy, switching between them at a leisurely pace. You may want to use the time to try some of the meditations suggested on these pages, or elsewhere in the book. Set aside time for talking and for sleeping or just lying in each other's arms. You should both feel recharged by your day. After your last meditation–or throughout the day–indulge in passionate lovemaking, enjoying the renewed feeling of closeness.

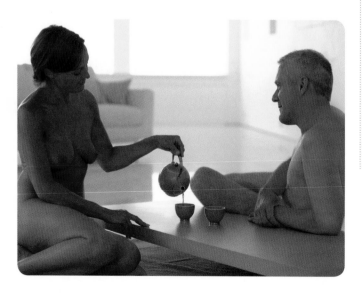

tantric tea ceremony

This ceremony is easy to set up and works well to help you engage deeply with your partner. For added sensuality, perform this ceremony naked, and compliment your partner on their beautifully relaxed body.

1 Sit opposite each other comfortably and namaste each other to begin (see page 10).

2 One partner pours the tea for the other, then holds the cup for at least three minutes. Look into the cup, and pour your essence into the tea. Allow all of the aspects of your nature to rise up and overflow into the tea.

3 Hand the tea to your partner, who drinks slowly, imagining your divine essence mixing and merging with his or her own essence.

4 Repeat the ritual the other way around, so the other partner can savor the ceremony.

5 Namaste to complete the meditation.

yin yang game

This game invites you to create the world of your fantasies, without compromise or dilution. If one or both of you are used to thinking mostly about the desires of others, this will be a useful challenge. In this game the partner in the role of "yin" is receptive and supportive, and the "yang" partner is determining and guiding.

1 Agree on how long you will devote to this game, from an hour to the rest of the weekend. Divide the time equally between you. When playing for the first time, ensure that each of you has more than one chance to be yang so you are able to grow in confidence.

2 The partner who is yang decides what you will do together, whether going out for a walk or asking for a sexual treat. Yin should support these wishes as much as possible. If you don't want to do something, seek an alternative together.

3 At first it may seem as if the yang role is the most exciting, but there are many pleasures to be found in the yin role. Enjoy not having to make any decisions, and learning to see

the world through your partner's eyes. This is a valuable chance to learn about your partner's desires, and to take pleasure in fulfilling them.

4 Use the game to explore your sexual fantasies. You may pretend that you are meeting for the very first time, or try some role-play. You could take erotic photographs of each other, or make love outdoors.

5 Yin is responsible for time keeping, but if yang's wish takes you away from home, make sure you plan to get back within the time allotted. If you need to discuss anything, stop the clock for a while, then resume once you are both happy with the next step in the game.

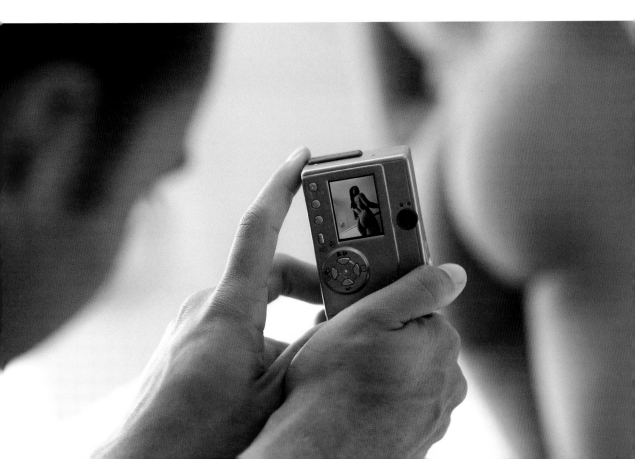

Day three

On your last day, recharge yourselves with time spent outdoors and in energetic physical activity. Absorb the beauty of your surroundings and the physical presence of your partner, so that these memories return home with you, as a continual source of rejuvenation.

a day of rejuvenation

As you emerge recharged from the relaxing activities of the previous day, you will be ready to increase your energy levels and enter a day of rejuvenation and celebration. Spend the last day of your retreat outdoors, engaging in simple but energetic activities such as walking in nature, taking in the beauty of your surroundings. As you move through nature, leave mundane concerns behind you and note the feeling of liberation. Breathe deeply and let natural energy expand within you. Relish your connection with nature and allow yourself to become fully, joyously rejuvenated.

☯ Eating in silence

When eating outdoors, try to appreciate the meal together in silence. Chew slowly, savoring the flavours and textures of the food, and immerse yourself fully in this sensual experience. Notice the feeling of silent connection that comes from sharing this peaceful ritual with your partner.

breathing in nature

If the weather is fine enjoy a walk in nature together. Take a blanket with you so that you can find a secluded spot in which to meditate.

1 Lie down close to your partner under the sky or a tree. Embrace and breathe easily, allowing your body to expand and relax.

2 Let the sounds of the birds and insects, and the smells of the flowers enter you through your awakened senses. Become one with universal life-force energy as you feel the flow of it rising from the earth and filling your body.

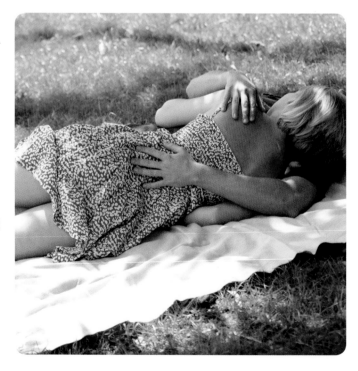

meditation of liberation

This is a wonderful way to end your weekend before you return home. This meditation is energizing and will leave you with a renewed sense of balance. Enjoy experiencing moments of rest and activity so close together, and make breath, dance, or rest your focus, depending on your energy level.

1 Stand opposite each other and visualize a spiral of energy coiling from your head down to your genitals.

2 Begin to dance wildly, feeling energy flooding up and down the spiral, waking up every cell in your body. With snakelike movements, let your body free itself. Make whatever sounds express your inner feelings.

3 Sit facing each other with your knees touching. Breathe in through your base chakra, allowing your breath to rise up and out of your second chakra. Imagine your breath fusing with your partner's, so that it becomes the shape of a helix.

4 Still sitting, sway and move your body, until you feel fully loosened. Breathe deeply, allowing your breath to expand and open your body and mind.

5 Breathe in through your second chakra and out through the third. Focus on your partner, letting your breaths merge. Move through each of the chakras, breathing in this way.

6 Feel the gathered energy at the crown of your heads. Allow it to expand throughout your body, flooding the chakra system all the way to your roots.

7 As you breathe out again, imagine the breath flowing down the front of your body, making a heart shape between you both. Expand the heart breath out to fill the room, then the building, country, planet, and universe.

8 Lie down together, holding each other's feet, to form a human yantra (see page 51). Continue softly with your breathing and let your bodies dissipate into bliss.

☺ Liberate your breath

Your breath comes from the very center of your being and is closely connected to your emotional states. You can often judge what a person is feeling by their breathing pattern. Quick surface breathing can tell you that a person is stressed, anxious, or nervous, while deep rhythmic breathing denotes a calm, steady, and relaxed state of mind. During lovemaking your partner's breathing pattern indicates his or her state of arousal and can therefore be arousing in itself.

Make it a point to listen closely to your partner's breathing as an insight into his or her emotional state. Notice the calm, steady way in which you are both breathing at the end of your retreat. Make a mental note of this feeling of relaxation and the atmosphere of the retreat. Later, you will be able to use your breathing to access a similar state of calm.

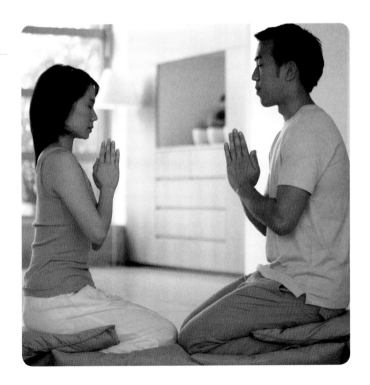

Returning home

As you return to the real world, make sure you tell your partner how much you have enjoyed your time together. Think also about how you can take the many benefits of your tantric weekend home with you, to serve as inspiration as you continue on your tantric journey.

acknowledging your partner

It's important to get into the habit of continually acknowledging your partner for the things you appreciate. In this way gratitude multiplies, naturally and unforced, and your partner flourishes in that love. This practice alone can transform a relationship.

Expressing positivity is a good habit to foster. As you return from your retreat, make it your priority to communicate to your partner how important he or she is to you. When you get home, write a letter to your partner, recording the moments that you will treasure. Mail or leave the letter for your partner to find. This will keep the experience alive for both of you, and serve as a tangible reminder of your gratitude. It will also remind you to plan another break away before too long.

meeting other tantric couples

One way to carry on the spirit of your retreat is to make an effort to meet others who practice tantra. This helps reinforce the tantric principles that you were able to focus on fully while you were away, and gives you a larger sense of the community you shared with your partner during your retreat.

Hearing how other couples are benefiting from tantra can be inspiring and motivating. It will help you both to realize that you're not the only couple who face challenges, and it can be profoundly empowering to talk openly with other couples about your sex life and the rituals you share.

A good way to meet other tantricas is to go on a couple's workshop. In a short space of time it can feel as if you've known the couples forever. You could also find tantric couples through local networks or organizations, and form a support group.

◈ Ways to acknowledge your partner

It is easy to take your partner for granted. Try one of these ways to show your partner how much you love and desire him or her:
- Start each day with a short meditation together, before you get out of bed.
- After a memorable evening or holiday, send a letter or note to thank your partner.
- Send a sexy text message or leave a note at home for your partner to find.
- Remember to thank your partner verbally for little things — a kind gesture, help given, or when they make you laugh.

the appreciation ritual

Practice this ritual regularly at home to strengthen and affirm your relationship. It will help create openness and intimacy. Try to see your partner as a mirror, and look to find the qualities in your partner that can help you to grow in yourself.

1 Sit together in your sacred space. Namaste each other to begin (see page 10).

2 Think of three things you especially love or admire about your partner. They don't have to be the three most important things.

3 The woman speaks first, telling her partner her three thoughts, and calling him by name: "John, what I love about you is…" Next, he speaks, calling her by name and using the same formal expression. Take your time and let the words resonate with the listener.

4 The woman then says: "John, what I would like you to teach me is…" He then does the same, using her name.

5 Finish with a namaste, then kiss and embrace, thankful for your partner's ability to share and praise openly.

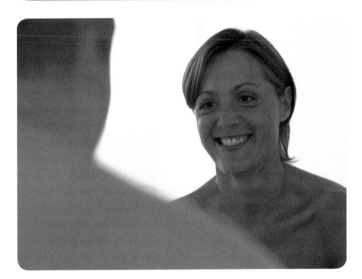

✆ Teach each other

An important part of tantra is learning from your partner. In the ancient tantric texts, the god Shiva is sometimes a teacher for Shakti. At other times, she teaches him, and he listens and asks questions with respect and thoughtfulness. In this way, you can learn and grow from each other's strengths.

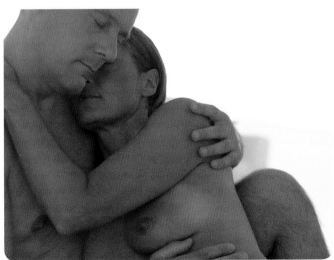

RESOURCES

BOOKS

Consult these books for inspiration and advice on sex, relationships, the body, and tantric practice. The erotic literature titles are especially good for spicing up your meditation time and provoking new fantasy scenarios.

tantric sex and love

Sex & Happiness
by Laurie Handlers
(Butterfly Workshop Press, 2007)

Tantric Love
by Ma Ananda Sarita & Swami Anand Geho (Gaia Books, 2005)

Tantric Quest
by Daniel Odier
(Inner Traditions, 1997)

Urban Tantra
by Barbara Carrellas and Annie Sprinkle
(Celestial Arts, 2007)

The Yoni
by Rufus C. Camphausen
(Inner Traditions, 1996)

sex techniques and massage

Erotic Massage
by Anne Hooper
(Dorling Kindersley, 2005)

Erotic Massage: The Touch of Love
by Kenneth Ray Stubbs
(Tarcher, 1999)

Naughty Tricks and Sexy Tips
by Dr. Pam Spurr
(Amorata Press, 2007)

health and wellbeing
Fire in the Belly: On being a man
by Sam Keen
(Bantam, 1992)

Perfect Health
by Deepak Chopra
(Bantam, 2001)

Sexual Ecstasy and the Divine
by Yasmin Galenorn
(Crossing Press, 2003)

The Way of the Superior Man
by David Deida
(Sounds True, 2004)

Women Who Run With the Wolves
by Clarissa Pinkola Estes
(Ballentine, 1996)

Women's Bodies, Women's Wisdom
by Dr. Christiane Northrup
(Bantam, 2006)

You Can Heal Your Life
by Louise Hay
(Hay House Inc, 1999)

erotic literature
The Claiming of Sleeping Beauty
by Anne Rice
writing as A.N. Roquelaure
(Plume, 1999)

Exit to Eden
by Anne Rampling
(Avon, 2007)

Men in Love
by Nancy Friday
(Delta, 1998)

Woman on Top
by Nancy Friday
(Pocket, 1993)

inspirational reading
In the Dark and Still Moving
by Anne Geraghty
(The Tenth Bull, 2007)

Excuse Me, Your Life is Waiting
by Lynn Grabhorn
(Hampton Roads, 2003)

WEBSITES

Use these websites to find information on tantra, personal blogs related to the tantric experience, general information about health and well-being, as well as a selection of classes and workshops.

Tantra Link
www.tantralink.com

Living Tantra
www.livingtantra.net

Human Awareness Institute
www.hai.org

FILMS

Erotic films are powerful sensual stimulants. If you and your partner do not already take advantage of this sexy form of entertainment, start with one (or more) of these overtly erotic and beautifully-shot selections.

Aria
(Studio A Entertainment, 2001)

Dollhouse
(Studio A Entertainment, 2003)

Nine Songs
(Revolution Films, 2005)

Shortbus
(Fortissimo Films, 2006)

HEALTH AND FITNESS

Detox regularly, either at home or at a retreat center, to lose weight, deal with any digestive problems, and increase your energy levels. Try 5 rhythms dance to learn classic rhythmic patterns, NIA dance to focus on holistic well-being, and Pilates to stretch, relax, and tone

detox treatments
Detox America
www.detoxamerica.com

Dr. Schulze's original clinical formulae
www.herbdoc.com

dance and exercise
5 rhythms dance
www.movingcenterschool.com

NIA dance
www.nianow.com

Pilates
www.pilates.com

RETREATS
Try one of these retreat locations—or a favorite local spot—to reconnect with your partner and yourself.

Rancho La Puerta
www.rancholapuerta.com

Institute for Ecstatic Living
www.ecstaticliving.com

Omega Institute
www.eomega.org

Osho Nisarga
www.oshonisarga.com

TANTRIC TOOLS
Search these well-stocked websites for meditation timers, blindfolds, a range of essential aromatherapy oils, floor seating options such as Back Jack chairs, and other tools and props for meditation.

e3
www.essentialthree.com

Floor seating
www.floorseating.com

Tantra.com
www.tantra.com

Mindfold
www.mindfold.com

Sound travels
www.soundtravels.co.uk

Gongtimers
www.gongtimers.com

MUSICAL RESOURCES
Experiment with different types of music as you practice tantra. The suggestions below are a good starting point for capturing emotion during specific meditations, and all are easily downloadable through iTunes or other music websites. For music with an overtly sensual flavor, look for songs from Dakini Records, a label that develops music with tantra in mind.

Love and hate list *see page 25*
"Qu'ran"
by Brian Eno and David Byrne
(Sire Records, 1981)

"Migrations"
by Baka Beyond
(Hannibal, 1998)

"Regiment"
by Brian Eno and David Byrne
(Sire Records, 1981)

"Mariama"
by Pape and Cheikh
(Real World Records, 2003)

Yin yang touch *see page 32*
"Travels"
by Pat Metheny
(ECM Records, 1991)

"Isa Lei"
by Ry Cooder and V.M. Bhatt
(Water Lily Acoustics, 1993)

Pillow beating *see page 39*
"Killing in the Name"
by Rage Against the Machine
(Epic, 1992)

Dancing for an invisible lover
see page 66
"Kidda"
by Natacha Atlas
(Nation, 1997)

"The Ritual"
by Al Gromer Khan
(New Earth, 1998)

Free up your pelvis
see page 74
"Natasha"
by Makyo
(Dakini Records, 2001)

Kundalini rising *see page 76*
"Garden"
by Lumin
(Hearts of Space, 2002)

"Chandini Chowk"
by MIDIval PunditZ
(Six Degrees, 2002)

Sexy stripping *see page 78*
"Fell in Love With a Boy"
by Joss Stone
(S-Curve, 2003)

"Ooh La Lah"
by Goldfrapp
(Mute Records, 2006)

"Rush Over"
by Marcus Miller
(PRA, 1994)

Embracing the other
see page 82
"Only Believe in Love"
by Luxia
(Hi-Note Music, 2008)

"The Ingredients of Love"
by Angie Stone
(J-Records, 2001)

Lion's play *see page 84*
"Takshaka"
by Makyo
(Dakini Records, 2001)

"Udu Chant"
by Micky Hart
(Rykodisc, 1991)

Sharing music *see page 100*
"Piano sonata no. 14 in C sharp minor"
by Beethoven (1801)

"Adagio for Strings"
by Barber (1936)

"Balance"
by Benjy Wertheimer
(Benjy Wertheimer, 2006)

"Raga Darbari Kanada: Alap and Jor"
by Hariprasad Chaurasia
(Nimbus, 1993)

Receiving touch
see page 102
"Prayer in Passing"
by Anoushka Shankar
(Angel, 2005)

Enter the caress *see page 105*
"Monsoon Point"
by Amelia Cuni and Al Gromer Khan
(New Earth, 1995)

Chakra touch *see page 106*
"Arc"
by Ishq
(Interchill, 2002)

Yin yang gazing *see page 110*
"End of an Era"
by David Helpling
(Spotted Peccary, 1996)

Dancing the divine
see page 112
"Qi Gong"
by Puff Dragon
(Dakini Records, 2005)

"One Day Deep"
by Praful
(N-Coded, 2003)

Circular breathing *see page 118*
"Blue Raga"
by Al Gromer Khan
(New Earth, 1998)

Chakra breathing *see page 120*
"Chakra Breathing"
by Osho & Kamal
(Orchard, 2000)

Kiss exploration *see page 124*
"El Hadra"
by Klaus Wiese
(Aquarius International, 1996)

Erotic massage
see pages 128, 131, 132, 134
"Yu"
by Ishq
(Interchill, 2002)

"Long Distance"
by Rick Cox
(Cold Blue, 2001)

"Tibet Part 2"
by Mark Isham
(Windham Hill, 1989)

"Tantra Drums"
by Al Gromer Khan
(New Earth, 1998)

Worshipping the wand of light
see page 138
"Skin as soft as moonlight"
by Makyo
(Waveform Records, 2001)

"Ghost Dancer"
by Gabrielle Roth
(Raven, 1993)

Masculine principle
see page 150
"Shaman's prayer"
by Gabrielle Roth
(Raven, 1993)

Greeting the goddess *see page 154*
"El Hadra"
by Klaus Wiese
(Aquarius International, 1996)

"Spacefunk"
by Puff Dragon
(Dakini Records, 2005)

Shiva shakti dance
see page 159
"Tantrika"
by Yang Makyo
(Dakini Records, 2001)

"Underworld"
by Praful
(N-Coded, 2003)

"La Illaha"
by Bharamji and Maneesh De Moor
(Blue Flame, 2005)

"Soar Angelic"
by Makyo
(Dakini Records, 2001)

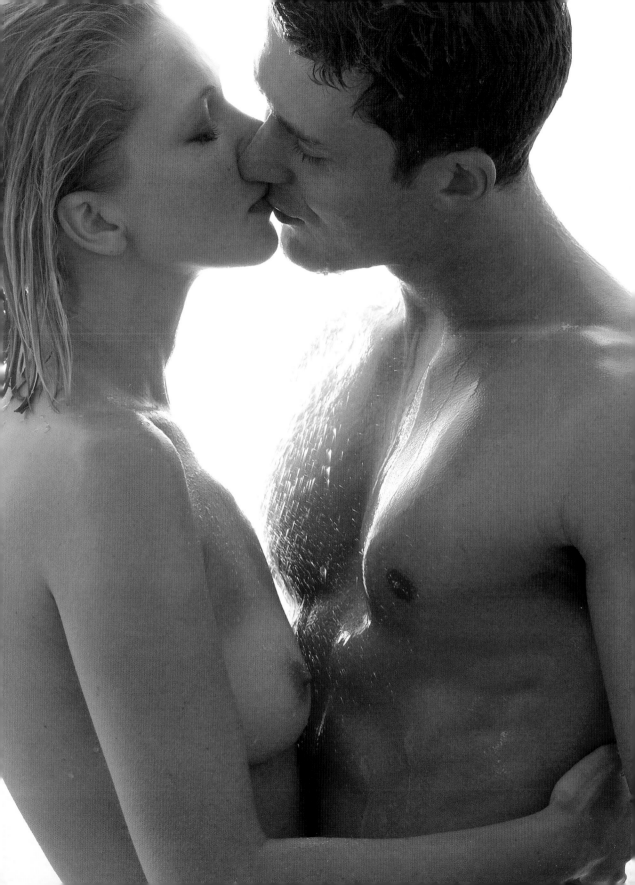

INDEX

ACKNOWLEDGMENTS

Author acknowledgments

I wish to dedicate this book to my beloved teacher and friend
Mahasatvaa Ma Ananda Sarita who has taught me many of these
meditations over the course of a joyful, ten-year training.
Many thanks go to:
Coco De Mer–for providing the glass dildo and
accoutrements on page 174.
John Hawken of Tantra Laboratory–for contributing
meditations for Yin Yang Touch, Yin Yang Game, and the
Appreciation Ritual.
Andrew–for teaching me so much about love.
Linda–for inspiration and guidance.
Claire Walmsley–for the kick start.
Samantha Richards–for seeing the possibility and getting the ball
rolling with your unique talent and savvy style.
John Glover – for artistic and emotional support throughout.

Jack Raymond–for your intelligence and regular doses of humor.
My friends–you know who you are. You also know how
I feel about you!
The Goddesses at Dorling Kindersley–for working with integrity, flair,
and above all, positivity.
Becky Alexander–for impeccable editing and patient hand-holding.
My mother and father–for believing in me always.
And last but not least, my two amazing boys–for the
unconditional love and acceptance.

DK acknowledgments

DK would like to thank Peter Mallory for his expert casting and
Alli Williams for on-set attention to make-up and hair. Thanks to
Marie Lorimer for indexing and Siobhan O'Connor for proofreading,
and to Laura Palosuo and Daniel Mills for their help with editorial.

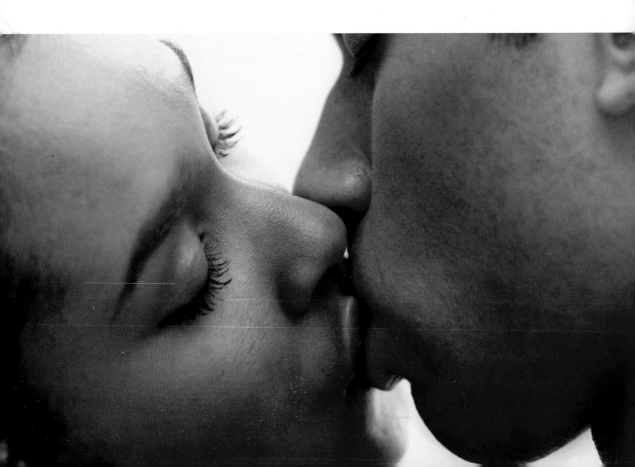